# Chronic Pain Management

*Editor*

DAVID T. O'GUREK

# PRIMARY CARE:
# CLINICS IN OFFICE PRACTICE

www.primarycare.theclinics.com

*Consulting Editor*
JOEL J. HEIDELBAUGH

September 2022 • Volume 49 • Number 3

**ELSEVIER**

1600 John F. Kennedy Boulevard • Suite 1800 • Philadelphia, Pennsylvania, 19103-2899

http://www.theclinics.com

**PRIMARY CARE: CLINICS IN OFFICE PRACTICE Volume 49, Number 3**
**September 2022 ISSN 0095-4543, ISBN-13: 978-0-323-98661-8**

Editor: Taylor Hayes
Developmental Editor: Jessica Cañaberal

*Primary Care: Clinics in Office Practice* (ISSN: 0095-4543) is published quarterly by Elsevier Inc., 360 Park Avenue South, New York, NY 10010-1710. Months of issue are March, June, September, and December. Periodicals postage paid at New York, NY and additional mailing offices. Subscription prices are $269.00 per year (US individuals), $672.00 (US institutions), $100.00 (US students), $312.00 (Canadian individuals), $696.00 (Canadian institutions), $100.00 (Canadian students), $368.00 (international individuals), $696.00 (international institutions), and $175.00 (international students). Foreign air speed delivery is included in all *Clinics* subscription prices. All prices are subject to change without notice. POSTMASTER: Send address changes to *Primary Care: Clinics in Office Practice*, Elsevier Periodicals Customer Service, 11830 Westline Industrial Drive, St. Louis, MO 63146. Customer Service Health Sciences Division, Subscription Customer Service, 3251 Riverport Lane, Maryland Heights, MO 63043. **Customer Service: 1-800-654-2452 (U.S. and Canada); 314-447-8871 (outside U.S. and Canada). Fax: 314-447-8029. E-mail: journalscustomerservice-usa@elsevier.com (for print support); journalsonlinesupport-usa@elsevier.com (for online support).**

*Reprints.* For copies of 100 or more, of articles in this publication, please contact the Commercial Reprints Department, Elsevier Inc., 360 Park Avenue South, New York, NY 10010-1710. Tel. 212-633-3874; Fax: 212-633-3820; E-mail: reprints@elsevier.com.

*Primary Care: Clinics in Office Practice* is covered in *MEDLINE/PubMed (Index Medicus)* and *EMBASE/ Excerpta Medica, Current Contents/Clinical Medicine,* and *ISI/BIOMED.*

# Contributors

## CONSULTING EDITOR

**JOEL J. HEIDELBAUGH, MD, FAAFP, FACG**
Clinical Professor, Departments of Family Medicine and Urology, Director of Medical Student Education and Clerkship Director, Department of Family Medicine, University of Michigan Medical School, Ann Arbor; Ypsilanti Health Center, Ypsilanti, Michigan

## EDITOR

**DAVID T. O'GUREK, MD, FAAFP**
Associate Professor and Interim Chair, Department of Family and Community Medicine, Lewis Katz School of Medicine at Temple University, Philadelphia, Pennsylvania

## AUTHORS

**ROBERT N. AGNELLO, DO, FACOFP**
Assistant Professor of Family Medicine, AOBFP Certified Family Medicine and Pain Medicine, Jerry M. Wallace School of Osteopathic Medicine, Campbell University, Buies Creek, North Carolina

**HIU YING JOANNA CHOI, MD**
Assistant Professor, Lewis Katz School of Medicine at Temple University, Philadelphia, Pennsylvania

**ROBERT L. "CHUCK" RICH Jr, MD, FAAFP**
Medical Director, Bladen Medical Associates, Elizabethtown; Clinical Adjunct Professor, Campbell University Osteopathic School of Medicine, Buies Creek, North Carolina

**SARAH COLES, MD, FAAFP**
Associate Professor, Department of Family, Community, and Preventive Medicine, University of Arizona College of Medicine-Phoenix, Phoenix, Program Director, Family and Community Medicine Residency, North Country Healthcare, Flagstaff, Arizona

**TRACEY CONTI, MD**
Chair, Department of Family Medicine, University of Pittsburgh School of Medicine, Pittsburgh, Pennsylvania

**WILLIAM DABBS, MD, FAAFP**
Assistant Professor, Family Medicine Clerkship Director, Department of Family Medicine, University of Tennessee Graduate School of Medicine, Knoxville, Tennessee

**KELLENE EAGEN, MD**
Assistant Professor, Department of Family Medicine and Community Health, University of Wisconsin Madison, Madison, Wisconsin

**SUSAN KUCHERA FIDLER, MD**
Clinical Assistant Professor of Family and Community Medicine, Sidney Kimmel Medical College, Philadelphia; Associate Director Family Medicine Residency, Abington Family Medicine, Jenkintown, Pennsylvania

**COREY FOGLEMAN, MD, FAAFP**
Deputy Director, Penn Medicine Lancaster General Health Family Medicine Residency Program, Lancaster, Pennsylvania

**GARETT FRANKLIN, MD, FAQSM**
Family Medicine and Primary Care Sports Medicine, Team Physician, North Carolina State University - Team Physician, Cary Medical Group, Cary, North Carolina

**NORA JONES, PhD**
Associate Professor, Department of Urban Health and Population Science, Associate Director, Center for Urban Bioethics, Lewis Katz School of Medicine at Temple University, Philadelphia, Pennsylvania

**REBECCA KELLUM, MD**
Fellow, Addiction Medicine Fellowship, University of Wisconsin Madison, Madison, Wisconsin

**MENACHEM J. LEASY, MD**
Assistant Clinical Professor and Program Director, Department of Family and Community Medicine, Lewis Katz School of Medicine at Temple University, Philadelphia, Pennsylvania

**ALEX MCDONALD, MD, FAAFP, CAQSM**
Department of Family and Sports Medicine Fontana California, Southern California Permanente Medical Group, Assistant Professor, Department of Family Medicine, Bernard J Tyson Kaiser Permanente School of Medicine, Fontana, California

**KATHRYN MCKENNA, MD, MPH**
Associate Director, Penn Medicine Lancaster General Health Family Medicine Residency Program, Lancaster, Pennsylvania

**DAVID T. O'GUREK, MD, FAAFP**
Associate Professor and Interim Chair, Department of Family and Community Medicine, Lewis Katz School of Medicine at Temple University, Philadelphia, Pennsylvania

**LAUREL RABSON, MD**
Fellow, VA Interprofessional Advanced Fellowship in Addiction Treatment, William S. Middleton Memorial Veterans Hospital, Madison, Wisconsin

**KATHLEEN REEVES, MD, FAAP**
Chair, Department of Urban Health and Population Science, Director, Center for Urban Bioethics, Professor of Clinical Pediatrics, Lewis Katz School of Medicine at Temple University, Philadelphia, Pennsylvania

**DANIEL SALAHUDDIN, MD, MPH**
Resident Physician, Department of Psychiatry, University of Pittsburgh Medical Center, Pittsburgh, Pennsylvania

**MARGOT LATRESE SAVOY, MD, MPH, FAAFP, FABC, CPE, FAAPL, CMQ**
Senior Vice President, Education American Academy of Family Physicians, Washington, DC; Associate Professor, Family & Community Medicine and Urban Bioethics & Population Health, Lewis Katz School of Medicine at Temple University, Philadelphia, Pennsylvania

**SUSANNE WILD, MD**
Associate Professor, Department of Family, Community, Preventive Medicine, University of Arizona College of Medicine–Phoenix, Phoenix, Arizona

# Contents

Chronic pain is a common presenting problem in primary care offices. Primary pain disorders and chronic pain secondary to another underlying medical problem can significantly impact a patient's function and quality of life. Chronic pain is a complex diagnosis requiring individualized biomedical, psychosocial, and behavioral evaluations for each patient. Through thorough patient interview, physical examination, diagnostics, and standardized assessment tools, primary care clinicians can create a robust care plan for patients with chronic pain. Given the multifaceted nature of chronic pain, it is a diagnosis that fits into chronic disease model of care managed appropriately in the primary care setting.

Pharmacologic management of chronic pain is one component of a patient-centered care plan. Multiple classes of medications are available and can be used individually or in combination. Choice of medication is determined by the type and cause of pain, safety profile of the medication, patient values and preferences, comorbid conditions, cost, and availability. Incorporating shared decision making is critical when implementing a pharmacologic pain management regimen.

With benefits on pain and pain-related outcomes and low-risk profile, there has been an emphasis on nonpharmacologic management of chronic pain. Physical therapy uses exercises, manual therapies, and electrotherapy. Exercises include aerobic, strengthening, and flexibility exercises. Aquatic exercises have similar efficacy to land-based exercises. Multidisciplinary care uses a biopsychosocial approach. All are effective for pain-related outcomes. Occupational therapy focuses on ergonomics, joint protection, orthoses, and assistive devices. Limited evidence exists for taping, orthoses, assistive devices, thermotherapy, and education on pain-related outcomes. Weight loss in patients who are overweight or obese is effective for pain reduction in knee arthritis.

treatment. An awareness of the stigma facing patients with both CNCP and SUD is important to providing compassionate, patient-centered care.

Chronic pain syndromes include chronic low back pain, tension type and migraine headaches, fibromyalgia, and osteoarthritis. Adjunctive therapies may provide real benefit by themselves, as well as when combined with one another and more traditional treatments such as medication and physical therapy. High-quality evidence, including systematic reviews, and/or clinical practice guidelines support the use of acupuncture, acupressure, massage, and/or mindfulness-based stress reduction (MBSR) in patients with one or more of these chronic pain syndromes.

Chronic pain is a significant public health concern. Care for patients with chronic pain is complex and involves many intersecting systems, policies, and procedures. Applying systems engineering concepts to chronic pain management opens the door to addressing a wide range of performance gaps through a structured, evidence-based approach. Successful implementation of systems-based practice includes effectively incorporating interprofessional teamwork, community resources, team-based care, patient safety, hospital readmissions, use of evidence-based medicine, transitions of care, and care for the underserved, including social determinants of health into the routine delivery of health care services including pain management.

Health care providers are ethically obligated to provide effective management for patients suffering from chronic pain. Many patients have not had access to such management, and current bioethical principles are not sufficient to create the roadmap needed on how to improve current standard of care. Principles described in the emerging field of urban bioethics greatly enhance the toolbox available to providers regarding chronic pain management. Redefining the principles of autonomy, beneficence/nonmaleficence, and justice to agency, social justice, and solidarity is essential to having the framework needed to provide more ethical, equitable care.

Rising rates of prescription opioids for chronic pain from the 1990s along with a concomitant worsening overdose crisis led to rapid evaluation and public health strategies to curb problems with prescription opioids. Guideline development, grounded in solid theory but based on limited evidence that translated into rigid and discordant policies, has contributed to controversies in pain management, worsening the treatment experience for people experiencing chronic pain and highlighting existing inequities from a system clouded with systemic racism. Newer public health approaches need to evaluate root causes and be more holistic addressing inequities as well as using trauma-informed principles.

# PRIMARY CARE:
# CLINICS IN OFFICE PRACTICE

---

**SERIES OF RELATED INTEREST**

*Medical Clinics* (http://www.medical.theclinics.com)
*Physician Assistant Clinics (https://www.physicianassistant.theclinics.com)*

---

**THE CLINICS ARE AVAILABLE ONLINE!**
Access your subscription at:
www.theclinics.com

# PRIMARY CARE:
# CLINICS IN OFFICE PRACTICE

## FORTHCOMING ISSUES

**December 2022**
Telehealth
Kathryn M. Harmes, Robert J. Heizelman, and Joel Heidelbaugh, Editors

**March 2023**
Behavioral Health
Meagan Vermeulen, Editor

**June 2023**
Allergy and Immunology
Andrew Lutzkanin III and
Kristen M. Lucassen, Editors

## RECENT ISSUES

**June 2022**
Diabetes Management
Lenny Salzberg, Editor

**March 2022**
Office-based Procedures: Part II
Karl T. Clebak and Alexis Reedy-Cooper, Editors

**December 2021**
Office-based Procedure: Part I
J. Lane Wilson and Jonathan Bridbord, Editors

## SERIES OF RELATED INTEREST

Medical Clinics: www.medical.theclinics.com
Physician Assistant Clinics: https://www.physicianassistant.theclinics.com

# Foreword
# "Suffer Not"

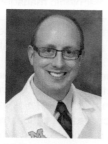

Joel J. Heidelbaugh, MD, FAAFP, FACG
*Consulting Editor*

Recently, I was explaining to one of my residents that when I was a medical student in the 1990s, I really don't remember learning about or seeing many patients who were treated for chronic pain management. During my family medicine residency, I remember when the Joint Commission on Accreditation of Healthcare Organizations mandated that clinicians must consider pain as the "fifth vital sign." At that point, pain assessments became ubiquitous, and not only did we recognize pain to a greater degree, but also we began to write many more prescriptions for pain medications, specifically opiates. Along came OxyContin, the touted "revolution in chronic pain management," and the number of prescriptions for all opiates (even methadone) skyrocketed. Hydrocodone-acetaminophen was the most widely prescribed generic medication for nearly a decade. In 2010, propoxyphene was withdrawn from the market due to risk of abuse and a Food and Drug Administration warning of potential cardiac toxicity. It has been stated that clinicians overprescribed controlled substance pain medications, which is likely an understatement.

And you all know what has transpired in the last decade. The Centers for Disease Control and Prevention ranks unintentional injuries as the leading cause of death in Americans up to 44 years of age, most of which are overdoses, yet we still have the challenges of managing chronic pain in our patients. While all of this has happened, many health care professionals have retreated in treating chronic pain with opiates, which has led to an overall decline in the number of providers who are willing to treat chronic pain at all. Unfortunately, this trend has led to an increase in patient suffering, a decline in their quality of life, and sometimes patients resorting to alternative means of pain management with devastating consequences. With the advent of targeted provider education coupled with easier access to pharmacy surveillance and monitoring systems, safe prescribing practices and therapeutic guidelines have paved the way for practices to better embrace these challenges.

Prim Care Clin Office Pract 49 (2022) xiii–xiv
https://doi.org/10.1016/j.pop.2022.07.002
0095-4543/22/© 2022 Published by Elsevier Inc.

primarycare.theclinics.com

This issue of *Primary Care: Clinics in Office Practice* takes a quantum leap forward in providing a cogent blueprint for clinicians to develop both comfort and skill in embracing chronic pain management in their practices. Articles highlight the history of chronic pain and its management, strategies for evaluation of patients with chronic pain, ethical challenges, and guidelines and policies. Experts provide the latest recommendations and evidence on pharmacologic and nonpharmacologic management of chronic pain, strategies for managing chronic pain in patients with substance abuse disorder, and even novel integrative strategies for care. Personally, I learned the greatest amount of new information from the article on trauma and behavioral health care for patients with chronic pain.

I offer my gratitude to Dr David O'Gurek, who did a phenomenal job as the guest editor of this issue in creating an impressive collection of articles centered on the management of chronic pain. I expect that this issue of *Primary Care: Clinics in Office Practice* will serve as a benchmark for both clinical practice and education, as it provides a wide scope of material for our readers that has not been presented in any current publication format. I also acknowledge the dedicated and knowledgeable authors who provided in-depth articles highlighting the current literature and guidelines. As with all of our issues of *Primary Care: Clinics in Office Practice*, we trust that this will serve as a go-to reference for daily practice. Most importantly, I hope that this issue bolsters our confidence to highlight to our patients that we understand their unique needs, and we can help them to not suffer.

Joel J. Heidelbaugh, MD, FAAFP, FACG
Departments of Family Medicine and Urology
Department of Family Medicine
University of Michigan Medical School
Ann Arbor, MI, USA

Ypsilanti Health Center
200 Arnet Suite 200
Ypsilanti, MI 48198, USA

*E-mail address:*
jheidel@umich.edu

# Preface

# Chronic Pain: Opportunities Amid Adversity

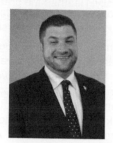

David T. O'Gurek, MD, FAAFP
*Editor*

Chronic pain, experienced by patients across the lifespan, is a common global health problem. The management of chronic noncancer pain remains a discomfort among clinicians, in part, due to limited scientific understanding of the pathophysiology as well as difficulty accessing the comprehensive, multidisciplinary programs and services that are cited as best practice. In addition, the experience of how best to provide care to a person and population that experiences significant morbidity and effects quality of life amid limited evidence, limited effective treatments, treatment guidelines codified into law that stipulates how one must practice can result in vicarious trauma for the treatment community.

This experience, however, in no way can compare with that of the individual sitting in the office in front of us confronted with chronic pain. In many ways, inequities and stigma regarding chronic pain have impacted this population and understandably created trust issues with patients and clinicians. Understanding these past challenges as well as confronting the reality of the difficulty with which to navigate care for patients experiencing chronic pain, primary care physicians have a unique role to play to deliver compassionate, patient-centered care even in the face of limited scientific understanding and treatment modalities.

Within this issue, you will find a wide breadth of topics focused on chronic pain, including evaluation, management, ethical and sociologic perspectives, systems-based practice, and the impacts of policy and public health. While not intended to be comprehensive, the authors shed light on core principles that can assist the primary care community in broadening perspectives on the biologic, psychologic, and social components that impact the health of individuals and populations experiencing chronic pain. Deeper discussions and partnerships between clinicians and patients, particularly in the advocacy realm, are certainly needed to make the essential policy changes to overcome the adversity. But, if we work together, we will go farther.

Prim Care Clin Office Pract 49 (2022) xv–xvi
https://doi.org/10.1016/j.pop.2022.07.001
0095-4543/22/© 2022 Published by Elsevier Inc.

primarycare.theclinics.com

It was an absolute pleasure working with an outstanding group of authors who contributed to this issue of *Primary Care: Clinics in Office Practice*. As we embarked on this journey, each of us learned more in the process, and our sincere hope is that this issue will provide you with similar educational advancement to provide quality care to our populations.

David T. O'Gurek, MD, FAAFP
Department of Family & Community Medicine
Lewis Katz School of Medicine
at Temple University
1316 West Ontario Street
Philadelphia, PA 19140, USA

*E-mail address:*
David.OGurek@tuhs.temple.edu

# Comprehensive Evaluation for Chronic Pain

Susan Kuchera Fidler, MD

## KEYWORDS

- Chronic pain • Assessment • Primary care • Standardized • Evaluation

## KEY POINTS

- Chronic pain is a complex diagnosis, and a comprehensive assessment should be conducted through interview, physical examination, indicated diagnostics, and standardized questionnaires.
- The assessment of a patient with chronic pain must address the individuality of each person's experience of chronic pain and should be conducted using a biopsychosocial approach.
- Correctly identifying the pain type or types experienced by a patient such as nociceptive, neuropathic, and central sensitization is important in developing a focused treatment plan.
- Multiple standardized assessment tools can assist in providing objective measures of pain intensity as well as patient function and quality of life.

## INTRODUCTION

Chronic pain is a common and important health issue impacting populations. Most conservative estimates suggest that 30% of people experience chronic pain at some point in their life, with some estimates as high as 50%.[1,2] Not only is the prevalence high but also the degree of impact on function and quality of life is profound. Many patients are unable to work and have multiple restrictions to participation in their daily life.[3,4] Patients with chronic pain are more likely to visit their primary care clinician as well as carry a higher overall illness burden.[2,4] The wide range of definitions used to describe chronic pain as well as the variability in pathology ranging from underlying intrinsic central nervous system disorders to pain attributable to specific pathology lend to a complex, multifaceted diagnosis.[5] Consequently, the assessment of chronic pain must entail an approach addressing the biomedical, psychosocial, and behavioral components relevant in providing care for a complex chronic disease. Primary care clinicians are uniquely positioned to provide holistic care for patients who experience chronic pain.

Abington Family Medicine, Sidney Kimmel Medical College, 500 Old York Road Suite 108, Jenkintown, PA 19046, USA
*E-mail address:* susan.fidler@jefferson.edu

Prim Care Clin Office Pract 49 (2022) 375–385
https://doi.org/10.1016/j.pop.2022.02.001
0095-4543/22/© 2022 Elsevier Inc. All rights reserved.

## DEFINITIONS

The definition of chronic pain lacks consensus. Yet, in our attempts to define pain, we start to understand the complexity of an individual's experience of chronic pain. In 2020, for the first time in 40 years, the International Association for the Study of Pain (IASP) revised their definition of pain to "An unpleasant sensory and emotional experience associated with, or resembling that associated with, actual or potential tissue damage" with further support that the experience of pain is specific to each individual with influences from biological, psychological, and social factors.[6] The Institute of Medicine defines chronic pain as pain that persists after one would expect the initial insult to have resolved and can exist with or without evidence of specific physical damage.[1] In terms of duration of how long the pain must be present, there also continues to be a variety of acceptable definitions. The IASP defines chronic pain as pain that "persists or recurs for more than 3 months" yet the National pain strategy defines chronic pain as "pain occurring on at least half the days for at least 6 months.[7,8] Although the definitions of chronic pain vary, in general the pain must persist for at least 3 months, provide an unpleasant experience for the patient, and may occur with or without any signs of overt physical damage.

As more is understood about the neurobiology of chronic pain, it has been accepted that chronic pain is a diagnosis unto itself, independent of the medical diagnoses that may contribute to the pain. The IASP and World Health Organization have further tried to classify chronic pain into primary chronic pain syndromes and secondary chronic pain syndromes.[7] This reclassification will allow International Classification of Diseases, 11th edition to reflect chronic pain as its own independent diagnosis that contributes to the complexity of a patient's overall health. Further classification will also assist clinicians in choosing therapeutics and modalities in the treatment of chronic pain. With these new diagnosis codes, pain related to a specific diagnosis can be coded to reflect that the pain is a separate complexity of the diagnosis. Chronic primary pain syndromes can include one or more areas and have significant emotional and functional impact. Chronic secondary pain can come under 6 types: cancer-related, postsurgical/posttraumatic, neuropathic, headache/orofacial, persistent visceral inflammation, and musculoskeletal pain.[2,7] See clinical examples listed in **Table 1**. Even though these classifications exist, many patients have overlapping chronic pain etiologies that do not always fit cleanly into one diagnostic category; this further supports the need for a whole-person assessment of chronic pain.

### *High-Impact Chronic Pain*

In 2016 the National Pain Strategy for population research began the task of improving the precision of how we define, prevent, treat, manage, and research pain with a population health focus. In the development of how to define chronic pain, it was clear that a subset of patients had a much higher burden of illness than other patients with chronic pain. This population was defined as high-impact chronic pain (HICP). These patients were defined as pain for more than 6 months with significant restrictions of life activities including work, social, leisure, and self-care.[8] In the United States, the prevalence of HICP approaches 5% of the population. These patients report increased pain severity, increased mental health diagnoses, greater use of health care resources, and greater challenges with self-care. Those with HICP were more likely to be female, older, have lower education, and have higher rates of divorce or separation. Patients with HICP were much more likely to carry other chronic health diagnoses, likely chronic obstructive pulmonary disease, kidney and liver disease, diabetes, asthma, and history of stroke. Furthermore, nearly 85% of this population was unable

**Table 1**
**International Association for the Study of Pain International Classification of Diseases 11th edition classification of chronic pain diagnoses**

| ICD-11 Diagnosis | Clinical Examples Causing Pain |
|---|---|
| Chronic primary pain | Fibromyalgia<br>Complex regional pain syndrome<br>Chronic migraine<br>Irritable bowel syndrome<br>Nonspecific low back pain |
| *Chronic secondary pain* | |
| Cancer-related pain | Due to cancer or treatment of cancer |
| Postsurgical/posttraumatic | Due to operative intervention or injury |
| Neuropathic | Diabetic neuropathy<br>Poststroke pain |
| Headache/orofacial | Cranial neuralgias<br>Dental pain |
| Persistent visceral inflammation | Inflammatory bowel disease<br>Vascular ischemia |
| Musculoskeletal | Rheumatoid arthritis<br>Osteoarthritis<br>Rigidity from spinal cord injury<br>Parkinson |

*Data from* Smith BH, Fors EA, Korwisi B, Barke A, Cameron P, Colvin L, Richardson C, Rief W, Treede RD; IASP Taskforce for the Classification of Chronic Pain. The IASP classification of chronic pain for ICD-11: applicability in primary care. Pain. 2019 Jan;160(1):83-87.

to work and was nearly 5 times more likely to access health care services.[9] In primary care, identifying patients who have HICP will allow clinicians to assist with accessing and supervising the multidisciplinary resources needed to support this patient population.

## ASSESSMENT

The experience of chronic pain is unique to an individual, and the assessment must represent that complexity. A comprehensive evaluation of chronic pain must include the biomedical, psychosocial, and behavioral health domains. Although a biomedical evaluation is warranted, this alone will not completely characterize a patient's pain because pain often exists without a biologically identifiable cause.[9] Using the biopsychosocial approach to chronic disease in the setting of chronic pain allows for identifying multidisciplinary treatment and management needs.[10] Pain must be assessed regarding physical impairment, magnitude of impact on daily function, and psychological or social factors that amplify the pain experience.[11] Through biological, social, and behavioral evaluations, the clinician can identify risk factors as well as protective factors that impact treatment and management.[12]

### Biomedical

Three main pain types are used to describe the experience of pain: nociceptive, neuropathic, and central sensitization. Nociceptive pain is defined by IASP as "Pain that arises from actual or threatened damage to non-neural tissue and is due to the activation of nociceptors."[13] Nociceptive pain is most often associated with tissue damage or inflammation and most often found in pain type with an underlying structural pathology.[13] Neuropathic pain is pain caused by disease of the nervous system and can be either central or peripheral. Long-standing nociceptive pain or neuropathic pain can create peripheral sensitization leading to allodynia and hyperalgesia often found in central sensitization.[14] Central sensitization exists without identifiable nerve or tissue damage and presents as general hypersensitivity to many stimuli.[5,14] Patients with central sensitization will often have contributing factors such as pertinent family history, history of physical or psychological trauma, and increased life stressors.[15] Clinical examples of each type of pain are noted in **Table 2**. However, many patients with chronic pain experience more than one type of pain, and some diagnoses overlap multiple types of pain (eg, complex regional pain syndrome). Classification of the pain type remains advantageous in selecting effective treatments.

### Psychosocial

A psychosocial assessment is critical in understanding a patient's experience of chronic pain. It has been shown that certain factors have a negative effect on the experience of chronic pain, whereas some offer a protective effect.[13] Identifying these factors is necessary in developing a multidimensional treatment program. Clauw and colleagues[12] described both psychosocial and behavioral health factors that led to increased vulnerability to chronic pain and factors that are associated with resilience in the experience of chronic pain (**Table 3**).[13] Additional psychosocial assessment should include a patient's physical functioning and physical activity, work and absenteeism history, interpersonal and caregiver relationships, sleep, and tendency toward pain catastrophizing.[13,16]

Pain-related disability is associated with decreased function and physical activity, and further, patients with chronic pain often overestimate the amount of physical activity they complete in a day.[17] Patients with chronic pain are less likely to work, and the severity of their pain is directly related to the amount of time spent working. Up to 20% of patients reported losing a job due to their chronic pain, and for those who continue to work, they show increase in rates of absenteeism, decreased productivity, and less social relationships at work.[18] This decrease in ability to work effectively also has a significant impact on a patient's finances and ability to contribute to household earnings and can lead to strain in interpersonal relationships.

Positive social support is associated with improved physical functioning for those with chronic pain, whereas having an unsupportive partner or family member is clearly related to poor chronic pain outcomes.[19] Owing to difficulty with physical activity, patients with chronic pain may restrict their leisure activities, including engaging with

| Table 2 | |
|---|---|
| **Clinical examples of pain types** | |
| **Type of Pain** | **Common Clinical Examples in Chronic Pain** |
| Nociceptive | Osteoarthritis, rheumatoid or inflammatory arthritis, central spine pain with pathology, gout, inflammatory bowel disease, chronic musculoskeletal pain (tendinopathies, ligament injury, and so on) |
| Neuropathic | Radiculopathy, diabetic neuropathy, postherpetic neuralgia, cranial neuralgias, pain s/p stroke or spinal cord injury, multiple sclerosis pain |
| Central sensitization | Fibromyalgia, irritable bowel syndrome, interstitial cystitis, tension headaches, chronic low back pain without pathology, phantom limb, vulvodynia |

| Table 3 Factors conferring increased severity of chronic pain and protective against worsening of chronic pain | |
| --- | --- |
| **Risk Factors** | **Protective Factors** |
| Trauma including physical, psychological, and sexual | Strong social and interpersonal relationships |
| Pain catastrophizing | Strong relationship with a psychotherapist |
| Sleep disturbance | Ability for adaptive coping and psychological flexibility |
| Pain-related fear | Mindfulness |
| PTSD or other mental health symptoms | Self-efficacy |

*Abbreviation:* PTSD, posttraumatic stress disorder.

*Data from* Clauw DJ, Essex MN, Pitman V, Jones KD. Reframing chronic pain as a disease, not a symptom: rationale and implications for pain management. Postgrad Med. 2019 Apr;131(3):185-198.

family and friends, unknowingly taking away a social support that may improve their experience of chronic pain. Caregivers also report high levels of stress in caring for patients with chronic pain and often report higher levels of anxiety and depression.[17,20] Given the ability of social supports to improve the course of chronic pain, a complete social history to help determine the patient's support system and to engage their support system in a complete treatment plan is needed.

Sleep disturbance is common for patients with chronic pain and clearly related to overall quality of life. The presence of sleep disorders in patients with chronic pain has been estimated to be near 50%, with specific difficulties in sleep initiation and maintenance.[21] Sleep disorders worsen subsequent experience of pain the following day, and increased pain creates poor sleep on the subsequent nights.[22] Assessing for sleep disorders provides another avenue to optimize a multimodal treatment plan for patients with chronic pain.

Finally, assessing a patient's thoughts, beliefs, and coping and resilience skills is critical to completing a thorough psychosocial evaluation. Specifically, clinicians should screen for pain catastrophizing, an exaggerated negative response toward chronic pain, including feelings of pessimism and helplessness. Catastrophizing has been specifically linked to increase in pain intensity, medication use, and medical care.[23] Despite its negative affect on pain, catastrophizing is responsive to behavioral therapy interventions, making it an essential component of a comprehensive chronic pain assessment.

### Behavioral Health

Mental health symptoms and diagnoses, including experienced trauma, posttraumatic stress disorder (PTSD), anxiety, depression, and substance use disorder, are common in chronic pain and are directly linked to increased intensity of pain, decreased function, increased use and misuse of opioids, and poor treatment response.[24–26] Furthermore, chronic pain is an independent risk factor for increase in suicide attempts and completions.[27] Patients have higher rates of both PTSD and anxiety, and often the anxiety is focused on the uncertainty of their chronic pain diagnosis.[28,29] Chronic pain and opioid use disorders (OUD) have what seems to be a bidirectional relationship with many patients with OUD having a chronic pain diagnosis that pre-dates their OUD diagnosis.[30] Appropriate identification of these mental health comorbidities is needed to optimize the management of chronic pain.

## OFFICE-BASED EVALUATION OF CHRONIC PAIN

The goal of the office evaluation of chronic pain is multifold: to evaluate for any intervenable or reversible causes of pain, to identify and quantify the type of pain experienced, and to evaluate for psychosocial and behavioral health factors that need to be addressed through a multidisciplinary treatment plan. This assessment should be completed through patient interview, physical examination, and diagnostics. Although consideration has been given to the use of standardized assessment tools, many have been created for use in clinical research and may not be easily applicable within the time and process constraints of outpatient care.

### Investigate for Intervenable or Reversible Causes of Chronic Pain

Standard history, physical examination, and tailored diagnostics should be part of the evaluation of chronic pain; this should be tailored based on the patient's specific pain complaints and working differential diagnoses. Yet among individuals with widespread pain, only a small percentage has a single definable diagnosis.[31] Clinicians should note that the degree of pain does not necessarily correlate with the identified pathologic condition.[10] The search for underlying pathologic condition should be undertaken separately from the patient's subjective pain reports. A physical examination appropriate for the pain complaint is important in identifying areas that may respond to treatments like physical therapy and identify red flag symptoms necessitating further evaluation. In addition to a focus physical examination, it is important for the clinician to assess pain behaviors present during the examination. The presence of pain behaviors such as grimacing, moaning, moving slowly, or rubbing the affected areas have been associated with increased pain intensity and overall disability.[32] Not all patients will require laboratory, imaging, or other diagnostic evaluations. It is important to review past records and to perform comprehensive laboratory tests, imaging, and diagnostic evaluations when appropriate.

### Identify Pain Type and Severity

As stated earlier, pain type is usually thought of as nociceptive, neuropathic, and central sensitization. Identifying both the type or types of pain and the intensity is critical in the pharmacologic management of chronic pain. Type of pain can be categorized through patient interview as well as several different standardized assessment tools. Patient reports of nociceptive pain are usually soreness, throbbing, aching, or cramping, whereas descriptions of neuropathic pain are more burning, stabling, pins and needles, or numbness. Central sensitization tends to be more widespread with features of allodynia and hyperalgesia but has more likelihood for mood and cognitive distortions as well as sensitivity to lights, noises, and smells. The ID Pain questionnaire uses 6 questions to differentiate nociceptive versus neuropathic pain with good accuracy.[33] Fibromyalgia, the representative form of central sensitization, has several screening and diagnostic standardized tools. However, the Fibromyalgia Survey, created by merging the Widespread Pain Index and Symptom Severity Score, not only identifies the patient with pain consistent with fibromyalgia but also may be useful in identifying general hypersensitization complaints.[34,35]

Pain intensity is often documented using validated single-dimension pain scales. The most used scales are the Numeric Rating Scale, Verbal Rating Scale, and Visual Analog Scale, which are all validated and reliable in clinical practice.[36] It is important to remember that these numeric intensity ratings will only represent a moment in time, which is insufficient in understanding chronic pain. Using these scales in a daily pain diary may be able to provide a better assessment of pain intensity over time.

Some standardized screeners will assess multiple domains like the frequently used short-form McGill Pain Questionnaire that evaluates pain type, location, and intensity.[37]

The assessment of function is critical in understanding the impact of chronic pain and areas for therapeutic intervention. Clinicians must assess the ability to complete Activities of Daily Living (ADLs) and instrumental Activities of Daily Living (iADLs) as well as ability to work, exercise, socialize, and participate in leisure activities. Clinical interview can help a clinician identify areas the patient may be struggling but is often subjective information that is difficult to track objectively over time. Although many general tools for assessing health-related quality of life exist (eg, Medical Outcomes Study, 36-Item Short-Form Health Survey), they can be long and difficult to introduce in clinical practice. The Pain Disability Index is a short 7-question screener that exists in the public domain evaluating function in home responsibilities, recreation, social

**Table 4**
**Selection of standardized assessment tools useable in clinical practice**

| Name of Standardized Tool | Description | Clinical Pearls |
|---|---|---|
| NRS | Pain intensity using a numbered scale like 1–10 or 1–100. | Easy and quick to use and track over time but only reflects one moment in time |
| VAS | Pain intensity measured by patient identifying pain intensity on the spectrum of a 100-mm line | Effective and can measure change in millimeter increments but more cumbersome to administer given need for actual 100-mm line and patient's ability to mark the line |
| VRS | Pain intensity using verbal descriptions like "mild," "moderate," "severe" | Easy to use but less room to reflect smaller changes over time given less response choices |
| ID Pain | Six-question screening tool to differentiate neuropathic pain from nociceptive pain | Easy to use in office practice but only consists of patient responses and should be correlated with physical examination findings |
| Fibromyalgia Survey | An assessment of widespread pain and somatic symptoms such as fatigue, sleep disturbance, and cognitive symptoms | Focused and short enough to use in office practice. Initially developed for fibromyalgia but may have applicability to pain due to central sensitization |
| Pain Disability Index | Seven-item scale examining the impact of pain in social and functional domains | Short, easy to apply in primary care, attempts to factor in function over time not just in the current moment |
| Brief Pain Inventory | Measures current and recent pain intensity and function as well as treatment effects | Useful for tracking pain and treatment response over time if completed at each visit |
| McGill Pain Questionnaire (short form) | Measures pain intensity, quality, and location. | The short form is easy to complete in an office appointment. It includes a 5-point VAS and the ability to locate pain via pictures |

*Abbreviations:* NRS, numeric rating scale; VAS, visual analog scale; VRS, verbal rating scale.

roles, work, sexual activity, self-care, and activities of daily living.[38] The Brief Pain Inventory (BPI) adds additional information by looking at pain intensity and function currently, over the past 24 hours, and a daily average to help put the patient's complaints at the visit in perspective to an average day.[39] **Table 4** summarizes a selection of standardized tools useable in a busy clinical practice.

### Evaluate Psychosocial and Behavioral Health Factors

Psychosocial factors are numerous and complex including thoughts, behaviors, and moods. A proposed screening acronym "ACT-UP" can assist the clinician in taking a psychosocial history. Clinicians should enquire about activities (including sleep and physical activity), coping, if they think their pain will improve, if they are feeling upset (anxious, depressed, and so on), and how people in their life respond to their pain.[12] Included in a psychosocial assessment should be the patient's goals for management of their chronic pain. Patient goals help clinicians provide whole-person care for what matters most to that individual; this is especially important because most standardized assessment tools do not often measure the outcomes most important to patients.[40]

Mental health diagnoses including depression, anxiety, PTSD, and substance use disorder should be addressed and uncovered during initial assessment of patients with chronic pain. Many standardized tools exist to screen for these mental health conditions, but the results can be difficult to interpret given the overlap in the somatic symptoms of chronic pain and other mental health diagnoses.[41]

### SUMMARY

Chronic pain is a complex diagnosis existing as a separate problem from the underlying diagnosis causing the pain. Primary care clinicians are ideally positioned to manage chronic pain given their expertise in the interplay of biomedical, psychosocial, and behavioral health factors in the patient's experience of chronic pain. A complete assessment of chronic pain should include an attempt to identify the contributing pain types (nociceptive, neuropathic, or central sensitization) as well as the impact of pain on their function and quality of life. Many standardized assessment tools exist to assist the clinician in collective objective and trackable data. Understanding the full extent of a patient's pain is the critical first step in a comprehensive, multidisciplinary treatment plan.

### CLINICS CARE POINTS

- Assessment of chronic pain must be undertaken with a biopsychosocial model in mind being sure to address all factors contributing to the patient's experience of chronic pain.
- Correctly identifying pain generators and pain types can be done through clinical interview or using standardized assessment tools like ID pain and the Fibromyalgia Survey and will impact treatment course selection.
- Standardized tools like the Pain Disability Index, BPI, and the short-form McGill Pain Questionnaire are all useable in clinical practice to assess pain intensity and impact on important life activities.

### DISCLOSURE

The author has nothing to disclose.

## REFERENCES

1. Institute of medicine, Committee on advancing pain research care, and education. In: Relieving pain in America: a blueprint got transforming prevention, care, education and research. Washington, DC: National Academy Press; 2011. Institute of Medicine.

2. Smith BH, Fors EA, Korwisi, et al. The IASP taskforce for the classification of chronic pain the IASP classification of chronic pain for ICD-11: applicability in primary care. PAIN 2019;18(1):83–7.

3. Taylor AM, Phillipps K, Patel KV, et al. Assessment of physical function and participation in chronic pain clinical trials: IMMPACT/OMERACT recommendations. Pain 2016;157(9):1836–50.

4. Pitcher M, Von Korff M, Bushnell MC, et al. Prevalence and Profile of high-impact chronic pain in the United States. J Pain 2019;20(2):146–60.

5. Stanos S, Brodsky M, Argoff C, et al. Rethinking chronic pain in a primary care setting. Postgrad Med 2016;128(5):502–15.

6. Raja SN, Carr DB, Cohen M, et al. The revised international association for the study of pain definition of pain: concepts, challenges, and compromises. Pain 2020;161(9):1976–82.

7. Treede RD, Rief W, Barke A, et al. Chronic pain as a symptom or a disease: the IASP classification of chronic pain for the international classification of diseases (ICD-11). PAIN 2019;160(1):19–27.

8. Department of Health and Human Services: National pain strategy: a comprehensive population health strategy for pain. Available at: https://www.iprcc.nih.gov/sites/default/files/documents/NationalPainStrategy_508C.pdf. Accessed on January 17, 2022.

9. Turk DC, Melzack R. Handbook of pain assessment. 3rd edition. New York, NY: Guilford Press; 2011.

10. Bevers K, Watts L, Kishino N, et al. The biopsychosocial model of the assessment, prevention, and treatment of chronic pain. US Neurol 2016;12(2):98–104.

11. Dansie EJ, Turk DC. Assessment of patients with chronic pain. Br J Anaesth 2013; 111(1):19–25.

12. Clauw DJ, Essex MN, Pitman V, et al. Reframing chronic pain as a disease, not a symptom: rationale and implications for pain management. Postgrad Med 2019; 131(3):185–98.

13. International Association for the Study of Pain. IASP terminology. 2018. Available at: https://www.iasp-pain.org/resources/terminology/. Accessed January 17, 2022.

14. Woolf CJ Central sensitization: Implications for the diagnosis and treatment of pain. Pain 2011;152:S2–15.

15. Bradley LA. Pathophysiologic mechanisms of fibromyalgia and its related disorders. J Clin Psychiatry 2008;69(S2):6–13.

16. Dueñas M, Ojeda B, Salazar A, et al. A review of chronic pain impact on patients, their social environment and the health care system. J Pain Res 2016;9:457.

17. Lerman SF, Rudich Z, Brill S, et al. Longitudinal associations between depression, anxiety, pain, and pain-related disability in chronic pain patients. Psychosom Med 2015;77(3):333–41.

18. Patel AS, Farquharson R, Carroll D, et al. The impact and burden of chronic pain in the workplace: a qualitative systematic review. Pain Pract 2012;12(7):578–89.

19. Meints SM, Edwards RR. Evaluating psychosocial contributions to chronic pain outcomes. Prog Neuropsychopharmacology Biol Psychiatry 2018;87:168–82.

20. West C, Usher K, Foster K, et al. Chronic pain and the family: the experience of the partners of people living with chronic pain. J Clin Nurs 2012;21(23–24): 3352–60.
21. Mathias JL, Cant ML, Burke AL. Sleep disturbances and sleep disorders in adults living with chronic pain: a meta-analysis. Sleep Med 2018;52:198–210.
22. O'Brien EM, Waxenberg LB, Atchison JW, et al. Intraindividual variability in daily sleep and pain ratings among chronic pain patients: bidirectional association and the role of negative mood. Clin J Pain 2011;27(5):425–33.
23. De Boer MJ, Struys MM, Versteegen GJ. Pain-related catastrophizing in pain patients and people with pain in the general population. Eur J Pain 2012;16(7): 1044–52.
24. Holmes A, Christelis N, Arnold C. Depression and chronic pain. Med J Aust 2013; 199(6):S17–20.
25. Kind S, Otis JD. The interaction between chronic pain and PTSD. Curr Pain Headache Rep 2019;23(12):1–7.
26. Feingold D, Brill S, Goor-Aryeh I, et al. The association between severity of depression and prescription opioid misuse among chronic pain patients with and without anxiety: a cross-sectional study. J Affect Disord 2018;235:293–302.
27. Racine M. Chronic pain and suicide risk: A comprehensive review. Prog Neuro-Psychopharmacology Biol Psychiatry 2018;87:269–80.
28. Siqveland J, Hussain A, Lindstrøm JC, et al. Prevalence of posttraumatic stress disorder in persons with chronic pain: a meta-analysis. Front Psychiatry 2017; 8:164.
29. Burke AL, Mathias JL, Denson LA. Psychological functioning of people living with chronic pain: A meta-analytic review. Br J Clin Psychol 2015;54(3):345–60.
30. Hser YI, Mooney LJ, Saxon AJ, et al. Chronic pain among patients with opioid use disorder: Results from electronic health records data. J Subst Abuse Treat 2017; 77:26–30.
31. Andersson HI, Ejlertsson G, Leden L, et al. Characteristics of subjects with chronic pain, in relation to local and widespread pain report: a prospective study of symptoms, clinical findings and blood tests in subgroups of a geographically defined population. Scand J Rheumatol 1996;25(3):146–54.
32. McCahon S, Strong J, Sharry R, et al. Self-report and pain behavior among patients with chronic pain. Clin J Pain 2005;21(3):223–31.
33. Portenoy R, Pain Steering Committee ID. Development and testing of a neuropathic pain screening questionnaire: ID Pain. Curr Med Res Opin 2006;22(8): 1555–65.
34. Wolfe F, Clauw DJ, Fitzcharles MA, et al. Fibromyalgia criteria and severity scales for clinical and epidemiological studies: a modification of the ACR Preliminary Diagnostic Criteria for Fibromyalgia. J Rheumatol 2011;38(6):1113–22.
35. Neville SJ, Clauw A, Moser SE, et al. Association between the 2011 fibromyalgia survey criteria and multisite pain sensitivity in knee osteoarthritis. Clin J Pain 2018;34(10):909.
36. Karcioglu O, Topacoglu H, Dikme O, et al. A systematic review of the pain scales in adults: which to use? Am J Emerg Med 2018;36(4):707–14.
37. Dworkin RH, Turk DC, Revicki DA, et al. Development and initial validation of an expanded and revised version of the Short-form McGill Pain Questionnaire (SF-MPQ-2). Pain 2009;144(1–2):35–42.
38. Pollard CA. Preliminary validity study of the pain disability index. Percept Mot Skills 1984;59(3):974.

39. Tan G, Jensen MP, Thornby JI, et al. Validation of the Brief Pain Inventory for chronic nonmalignant pain. J Pain 2004;5(2):133–7.
40. Gardner T, Refshauge K, McAuley, et al. Patient led goal setting in chronic low back pain—What goals are important to the patient and are they aligned to what we measure? Patient Educ Couns 2015;98(8):1035–8.
41. Harris CA, Joyce LD. Psychometric properties of the Beck Depression Inventory-(BDI-II) in individuals with chronic pain. Pain 2008;137(3):609–22.

# Pharmacologic Management of Chronic Pain

Sarah Coles, MD, FAAFP[a],*, William Dabbs, MD, FAAFP[b], Susanne Wild, MD[c]

## KEYWORDS

- Chronic pain • Pharmacotherapy • Pain management • Opioid • Neuropathic pain

## KEY POINTS

- Pharmacologic treatment should focus on the lowest effective dose for symptom relief and functional improvement while minimizing side effects and adverse events from pharmacotherapy.
- Medications can be used as monotherapy or combination therapy as a part of a multimodal pain management plan.
- Nonsteroidal anti-inflammatory drugs have significant side effects and should only be used for a limited time or if other therapies have failed.
- Anticonvulsants and antidepressants are first-line therapy for neuropathic pain.
- Opioids should be considered after exhausting other options for the treatment of chronic nonmalignant pain owing to significant risks.

## INTRODUCTION

Chronic pain is a complex issue with significant impacts on an individual's physical, emotional, and social health. Chronic pain can develop from diverse mechanisms, including underlying medical conditions, damaged tissue, and diseases of the somatosensory nervous system. The experience of chronic pain can vary dramatically between individuals and is shaped by attitudes, mood, belief systems, psychosocial, and socioeconomic factors. This wide variety of causes and experiences of pain can create challenges for the treating clinician. Pharmacologic management of chronic pain is one component of a multimodal, patient-centered care plan to address pain symptoms, improve function, and increase quality of life.

[a] Department of Family, Community, and Preventive Medicine, University of Arizona College of Medicine- Phoenix, Family and Community Medicine Residency, North Country Healthcare, 2920 North Fourth Street, Flagstaff, AZ 86004, USA; [b] Department of Family Medicine, University of Tennessee Graduate School of Medicine, 1924 Alcoa Highway, Box U-67, Knoxville, TN 37920, USA; [c] Department of Family, Community, and Preventive Medicine, University of Arizona College of Medicine–Phoenix, 1300 North 12th Street, Suite 605, Phoenix, AZ 85006, USA
* Corresponding author.
E-mail address: swhitley@email.arizona.edu
Twitter: @sarahmwc (S.C.); @billdabbs (W.D.); @susanne_wild (S.W.)

Prim Care Clin Office Pract 49 (2022) 387–401
https://doi.org/10.1016/j.pop.2022.01.005
primarycare.theclinics.com
0095-4543/22/© 2022 Elsevier Inc. All rights reserved.

There are multiple classes of pharmacotherapy used in the treatment of chronic pain. These include acetaminophen, oral nonsteroidal anti-inflammatory medications (NSAIDs), topical medications, muscle relaxers, anticonvulsants, antidepressants, and opioids. Pharmacologic treatment can be used as monotherapy or in combination. Pharmacologic treatment should focus on the lowest effective dosage for symptom relief and functional improvement, minimizing side effects, and consider comorbid conditions. This article discusses common classes of pharmacologic therapy for chronic pain, including considerations for use, efficacy, and safety.

## PHARMACOLOGIC CLASSES
### Acetaminophen

Acetaminophen is a centrally acting analgesic, whose mechanism of action is not fully understood. Acetaminophen is commonly used and available in a variety of preparations, many of which are readily accessible in over-the-counter products, making this a frequent first choice for many clinicians.

Unfortunately, the evidence of efficacy of acetaminophen in chronic pain syndromes is low.[1] Acetaminophen has not been shown to improve pain or function in osteoarthritis.[1] There are also no good studies to confirm efficacy in the management of neuropathic pain.[2] The 2021 National Institute for Health and Care Excellence guidelines for the management of chronic pain in individuals over 16 years old recommend against starting acetaminophen for chronic pain management. For patients already on this medication, it is recommended to discuss the lack of evidence to support the use of this medication, monitor for safety and efficacy, and explain risks.[3] This medication is most appropriately used for acute flares or when alternative medications are contraindicated.

The recommended maximum dosage of acetaminophen is 4 g a day. Although safe at recommended dosages, acetaminophen is also the most common cause of drug-induced hepatitis in the United States.[4] Some experts have recommended a maximum dose of 3 g a day when used chronically, even in the absence of other risk factors.[5] Because several over-the-counter drug combinations contain acetaminophen, patient education becomes important to avoid inadvertent medication overdose.

For patients with hepatic insufficiency, acetaminophen can be used in a case-by-case setting. Lowering the dosage to a maximum of 2 g/d appears to be safe and well tolerated in patients with chronic liver disease or cirrhosis.[6] Contraindications to acetaminophen include severe hepatic impairment and severe active liver disease, which could include decompensated cirrhosis, encephalopathy, and significant laboratory abnormalities. Other contributing factors, such as active use of alcohol, malnutrition, or chronic use of other medications, which interact with acetaminophen metabolism, need to be taken into consideration.[5]

### Nonsteroidal Anti-Inflammatory Medications

NSAIDs work by inhibiting cyclooxygenase, thereby reducing synthesis of prostaglandins and thromboxane. Although commonly used in the setting of acute pain and inflammation, NSAIDs have a role in chronic pain control as well. Unfortunately, their side-effect profile and associated risks limit their long-term use. This class of medications is most appropriately used as a short-term adjunct in the setting of an acute-on-chronic flare or injury, or if other therapies have failed.[7]

There is a long list of commercially available NSAIDs available in the United States. Their overall efficacy is often comparable in studies[8]; however, varied mechanisms of action, pharmacodynamics, metabolism, as well as pharmacogenetic factors play a

**Table 1**
**Nonsteroidal anti-inflammatory medications**

| Medication | Usual Dosage for Pain Management | Other Considerations |
|---|---|---|
| **Propionic acids** | | |
| Flurbiprofen | 50 mg 4 times a day or 100 mg twice or 3 times a day | |
| Ibuprofen | 200–400 mg every 4–6 h | Doses more than 400 mg rarely better for pain relief. Maximum daily dosage: 1200 mg |
| Ketoprofen | 75 mg 3 times a day or 50 mg 4 times a day | No substantial pain relief increase for dosage beyond 75 mg. Extended-release option available |
| Naproxen | 250–500 mg twice a day | Extended-release option available for once daily dosing |
| Oxaprozin | 600–1200 mg daily | Divided dosage may improve drug tolerance |
| **Acetic acids** | | |
| Diclofenac | 50 mg twice or 3 times a day | Extended-release option available |
| Etodolac | 200–400 mg every 6–8 h | Maximum daily dosage: 1000 mg |
| Indomethacin | 25–50 mg twice or 3 times a day | Extended-release option available |
| Sulindac | 150–200 mg twice daily | Association with hepatic inflammation and rare fatal hepatitis. Maximum daily dosage: 400 mg |
| Tolmetin | 400–600 mg 3 times a day | Maximum daily dosage: 1800 mg |
| **Oxicams** | | |
| Meloxicam | 5–15 mg once daily | |
| Piroxicam | 20 mg once daily | Medication has a long half-life; full effect may take 7–12 d after start of therapy |
| **Fenamates** | | |
| Meclofenamate | 50–100 mg every 4–6 h | LFTs need to be monitored in long-term use |
| **Nonacidic** | | |
| Nabumetone | 1000 mg once to twice daily | Active metabolite depends on biotransformation in the liver |
| **Selective COX-2 inhibitors** | | |
| Celecoxib | 200 mg once daily or 100 mg twice daily | Decreased GI side effects compared with other NSAIDs |
| **Salicylates** | | |
| Magnesium salicylate | 1160 mg twice daily | Monitor magnesium if using high doses |
| Diflunisal | 500 mg twice daily | |
| Salsalate | 1500 mg twice daily | Administer with food and large quantity (240 mL) of water or milk |

Usual dosage and other considerations for NSAIDs organized by type.
*Abbreviations*: COX, cyclooxygenase; GI, gastrointestinal; LFT, liver function tests.

role in selection for the individual patient (**Table 1**).[9] For example, reducing dosing frequency will lead to better medication adherence, but drugs with longer half-lives may be contraindicated for an elderly patient.

Given the longitudinal nature of chronic pain management, it is important to reevaluate patient risk factors on an ongoing basis, to assure that use of this class of medications is not contraindicated.[9] Other than hypersensitivity, absolute contraindications to chronic NSAID use include active peptic ulcer disease, chronic kidney disease, recent myocardial infarction, use after coronary artery bypass grafting, and severe heart failure. NSAID use should be avoid in the third trimester of pregnancy.[10]

In the setting of neuropathic pain, there is no good evidence for the efficacy of NSAIDs.[11] NSAIDs show a small magnitude of improvement in pain and disability for chronic low-back pain.[8] There is some evidence for improved pain and function in the intermediate and long-term treatment of osteoarthritic pain as well as inflammatory arthritis.[1]

## Topical Medications

### Transdermal nonsteroidal anti-inflammatory drugs

Topical NSAIDs are a good alternative to their systemic counterpart. Their mechanism of action is the same, but owing to decreased systemic absorption, adverse effects are less common. Topical ketoprofen and diclofenac have good evidence for efficacy in chronic pain. Topical NSAIDs are particularly useful for osteoarthritic pain, with numbers needed to treat of 6.9 for topical ketoprofen and 9.8 for topical diclofenac to achieve significant pain reduction.[12] There is no good evidence for the management of other sources of chronic pain.[12]

Although topical NSAIDs are a safer option, contraindications to use exist. Besides hypersensitivity to drug components, their use is limited on damaged skin. They also should be avoided in the setting of coronary artery bypass graft as well as advanced renal disease.[5] Oral NSAIDs and topical NSAIDs should not be combined, as there is increased risk of adverse events without evidence of increased efficacy.[13]

### Lidocaine

Lidocaine acts by blocking the initiation and conduction of nerve impulses. Topical preparations come in a variety of different delivery methods, including creams, patches, sprays, solutions, and ointments. Patches are easier to use than creams and gels and can be obtained over the counter at a concentration of 4%. Patches should be applied for no more than 12 hours in a 24-hour period. There is some evidence that topical lidocaine may be of benefit in the treatment of neuropathic pain, but generally the studies are of poor quality for chronic pain.[14] Some patches are Food and Drug Administration approved in the United States for the treatment of postherpetic neuralgia. Data are even more limited for chronic osteoarthritic pain.[14] Given the lack of systemic absorption and low likelihood of systematic adverse events, topical lidocaine could be considered for first-line treatment, especially in patients with other comorbidities that limit the use of alternative agents.[14] Patients should be cautioned against using occlusive dressings covering creams or gels owing to case reports of systemic toxicity, including seizure, arrhythmia, and death.[13]

### Capsaicin

Topical capsaicin works through a process of nociceptor defunctionalization. Preparations include a variety of different delivery methods, with different strengths. Studies have shown beneficial effect for the treatment of neuropathic pain with concentrations of 8%, delivered by a patch administered in the hospital or clinic setting out of concern for side effects (the number needed to harm for local pain was 16).[15] However, a single application can provide pain relief for up to 3 months.[16] The number needed to treat to reduce pain by at least half for patients with postherpetic neuralgia was 11.[15]

Lower concentrations of capsaicin must be applied 3 to 4 times a day and are available over the counter. Unfortunately, there is less evidence for their efficacy in either neuropathic or musculoskeletal pain.[17] For low concentrations of capsaicin, side effects are usually limited to local skin reactions that resolve upon cessation of product use.[13]

## Anticonvulsants

The anticonvulsants are commonly used to treat chronic pain syndromes. Frequently used anticonvulsants include gabapentin, pregabalin, carbamazepine, and oxcarbazepine. Gabapentin and pregabalin bind to the voltage-gated calcium channels in the central nervous system (CNS). However, the exact mechanism of action leading to pain improvement is unclear and seems to inhibit the release of excitatory neurotransmitters. Antiepileptic drugs like carbamazepine and oxcarbazepine might reduce conductance in sodium channels and inhibit nervous system ectopic discharges.

Anticonvulsant medications are recommended as a first-line therapy for neuropathic pain.[18] Pregabalin and gabapentin can reduce pain for individuals with neuropathic pain syndromes and have been demonstrated to improve function in individuals with fibromyalgia. These medications may also improve sleep compared with placebo for individuals with neuropathic pain.[1] Pregabalin has a more predictable dose response and a narrower therapeutic window and can be titrated more quickly than gabapentin.[19] Gabapentinoids have potential for euphorigenic effects at high or supratherapeutic doses, particularly when combined with opioids.[20] There is concern for potential misuse and abuse, and this risk appears highest for individuals with substance use disorder or concurrently taking opioids. Clinicians should be cautious when prescribing these medications and monitor for appropriate use, efficacy, and adverse events. Caution should also be taken when prescribing pregabalin or gabapentin in combination with other medications that have CNS depressing effects or for individuals with respiratory risk factors.[21]

Carbamazepine and oxcarbazepine are also used in some pain syndromes. Carbamazepine is the first-line treatment for trigeminal neuralgia, and oxcarbazepine is an alternative for individuals who cannot tolerate carbamazepine. Oxcarbazepine may also reduce pain severity for individuals with diabetic peripheral neuropathy but does not consistently improve quality of life.[1]

Anticonvulsants can have significant side effects as well as interactions with other medications. Medication choice should consider the safety profile in relation to the individual's comorbid conditions and risk factors (**Table 2**).

## Antidepressants

There are multiple classes of antidepressants used to treat chronic pain. These include tricyclic antidepressants (TCAs) and serotonin-norepinephrine reuptake inhibitors (SNRIs). Selective serotonin reuptake inhibitors are not as effective as other antidepressants in the management of chronic pain. The analgesic effects of antidepressant medications occur even in the absence of clinical depression and typically with lower doses than are required to treat depressive disorders. TCAs are thought to affect pain transmission by inhibiting reuptake of serotonin and norepinephrine in the descending pain pathways. TCAs also have histamine H1 receptor affinity. SNRIs inhibit both serotonin and norepinephrine without interference with the other neurotransmitters that may result in the TCA anticholinergic adverse effects.

**Table 2**
Anticonvulsants for chronic pain

| Medication | Dosage | Indications | Side Effects | Other Considerations |
|---|---|---|---|---|
| Pregabalin | Typical effective dose 150–600 mg/d in 2 or 3 divided doses | Peripheral neuropathy, postherpetic neuralgia, fibromyalgia | Peripheral edema, weight gain, xerostomia, dizziness, drowsiness, vision changes | Doses >600 mg/d increase side effects without additional benefit<br>Must be renally dosed. ER formulation not recommended in severe renal impairment |
| Gabapentin | Typical effective range 1200–2400 mg/d, with maximum dose of 3600 mg. Dose divided 3 times daily. Typical starting dose of 300 mg at bedtime | Peripheral neuropathy, postherpetic neuralgia, fibromyalgia | Dizziness, drowsiness, respiratory depression, peripheral edema, weight gain | Avoid use in myasthenia gravis (may exacerbate)<br>Must be renally dosed<br>Tolerance and dependence may develop<br>Should be tapered to avoid withdrawal symptoms |
| Carbamazepine | Typical maintenance dose 600–800 mg/d; maximum daily dose 1.2 g/d | Trigeminal neuralgia, glossopharyngeal neuralgia | Dizziness, drowsiness, ataxia, nausea, vomiting, speech disturbance, hypertension | Stevens-Johnson, toxic epidermal necrolysis, aplastic anemia, and agranulocytosis have been reported<br>If chronic therapy, taper over 2–6 mo to prevent withdrawal symptoms |
| Oxcarbazepine | 300–600 mg/d with maximum dose 1.8 g/d | Trigeminal neuralgia | Dizziness, drowsiness, headache, ataxia, fatigue, abnormal gait, vertigo, vomiting, abdominal pain, tremor, visual disturbance | Should be avoided in older adults owing to hyponatremia and SIADH risk<br>Must be renally dosed if CrCl <30 mL/min |

Common dosage, indications, side effects, and other considerations for anticonvulsant medications used in chronic pain. This is not meant to be an exhaustive list.
*Abbreviations:* CrCl, creatinine clearance; ER, extended release; SIADH, syndrome of inappropriate secretion of antidiuretic hormone.
*Data from* Refs.[1,19,34]

TCAs and SNRIs are recommended as a potential first-line therapy for neuropathic pain (**Table 3**).[18] TCAs are inexpensive and are often considered for use of associated pain-related insomnia. TCAs may reduce pain and improve sleep for individuals with fibromyalgia, but evidence is currently insufficient to draw firm conclusions.[1] TCAs did not demonstrate benefit in chronic low-back pain or HIV neuropathy.[4] Most studies evaluated amitriptyline, but the secondary amines, nortriptyline and desipramine, are often better tolerated owing to fewer anticholinergic effects.[19]

Commonly used SNRIs include duloxetine and venlafaxine. Duloxetine demonstrated small improvements in pain, quality of life, and function compared with placebo in neuropathic pain and osteoarthritis.[1] Duloxetine has also demonstrated small improvements in pain in chronic low-back pain. The number needed to treat for duloxetine to reduce pain 30% to 50% in patients with diabetic neuropathy was approximately 4 to 11.[22] Venlafaxine is less studied than duloxetine but may be a reasonable alternative if duloxetine is not available.

Of note, antidepressants can increase the risk of suicidal thinking and behaviors in children, adolescents, and adults. Individuals started on antidepressant medications should be monitored for suicidal ideation and provided appropriate resources to manage symptoms if they arise.

## Muscle Relaxants

Skeletal muscle relaxants are considered for use in chronic pain syndromes associated with spasticity, muscle spasms, and myofascial pain. Commonly used medications include centrally acting agents (such as methocarbamol), TCA-like agents (such as cyclobenzaprine), GABA-agonist agents (such as baclofen), and alpha-2 adrenergic agonists (such as tizanidine). In general, benzodiazepines do not play a role in chronic pain management. Psychological and physical functioning may be harmed by benzodiazepine use, and the addictive potential with this class of medication is a serious concern.[3] The metabolite of carisoprodol is sedating and has addictive potential, so carisoprodol is also not recommended.[18] Although there is some evidence of efficacy in acute musculoskeletal pain disorders, the efficacy of muscle relaxant medications is not well established in many chronic pain syndromes.[23] For example, most recent studies call into question the utility of muscle relaxants for chronic low-back pain.[24]

If clinicians use muscle relaxant medications, they should be cautious about adverse effects (such oversedation and CNS depression) as well as the risk of concomitant use with other sedating drugs or medications.

## Opioid Analgesics

The opioids represent a complicated class of analgesics that act as opioid receptor agonists. Although they have potent analgesic properties, their narrow therapeutic window limits the use of this class of medications. There are many indications for their use in acute pain settings, but there is potential for abuse, addiction, and dependence even with the shortest duration of prescriptions.[25] Those risks persist with chronic use. Although once considered first-line therapy for many chronic pain conditions, they are now widely discouraged for use in the treatment of chronic, nonmalignant pain and should be used as a last line.[26] Deleterious side effects are listed in **Box 1** and notably include constipation, respiratory depression, and death.[27]

Shared decision making should be used with patients to outline the appropriate risks and benefits of using this class of medications while incorporating the patient's perspective and preferences (see **Box 1**). If a clinician is considering prescribing an

**Table 3**
**Antidepressants for chronic pain**

| Class | Medication | Dosage | Indications | Side Effects | Other Considerations |
|---|---|---|---|---|---|
| TCA | Amitriptyline | 10–25 mg increased up to 150 mg at bedtime | Neuropathic pain, fibromyalgia, postherpetic neuralgia, migraine prevention, interstitial cystitis | Confusion, dizziness, drowsiness, cardiac dysrhythmia, xerostomia, vision disturbance, ataxia, urinary retention | Tertiary amines have greater anticholinergic effects and should be avoided in elderly |
| | Desipramine | 25 mg daily increased up to 150 mg/d | Diabetic neuropathy, postherpetic neuralgia | Confusion, dizziness, drowsiness, cardiac dysrhythmia, xerostomia, vision disturbance, ataxia, urinary retention | Secondary amines have fewer anticholinergic effects |
| | Nortriptyline | 25 mg daily increased up to 150 mg/d | Chronic low-back pain, diabetic neuropathy, myofascial pain, postherpetic neuralgia | Confusion, dizziness, drowsiness, cardiac dysrhythmia, xerostomia, vision disturbance, ataxia, urinary retention | Secondary amines have fewer anticholinergic effects |
| SNRI | Duloxetine | 20–60 mg once or twice daily | Diabetic neuropathy, fibromyalgia, osteoarthritis, chronic low-back pain, chemotherapy-related neuropathy | Nausea, dry mouth, constipation, dizziness, insomnia | Less insomnia than venlafaxine |
| | Venlafaxine | 37.5 mg daily increased to 150–225 mg daily | Diabetic neuropathy, fibromyalgia | Nausea, dry mouth, constipation, dizziness, insomnia | Less nausea than duloxetine |

Common dosage, indications, side effects, and other considerations for antidepressant medications used in chronic pain. This is not meant to be an exhaustive list.
*Data from* Refs. [1,19,34]

---

**Box 1**
**Side effects of opioids**

Common side effects of opioids
  Overdose
  Tolerance
  Physical dependence
  Increased sensitivity to pain
  Constipation
  Nausea and vomiting
  Dry mouth
  Sleepiness
  Dizziness
  Confusion
  Depression
  Low levels of testosterone
  Itching
  Sweating

*Adapted from* The Centers for Disease Control and Prevention. Prescription Opioids. 2017. Accessed October 27, 2021. https://www.cdc.gov/opioids/basics/prescribed.html.

---

opioid, they should familiarize themselves with their local and national guidelines and regulations to ensure legal and licensing compliance. All opioids outside of lower doses of codeine are schedule II drugs according to the US Drug Enforcement Agency (DEA). These drugs are defined as those with a "high potential for abuse, with use potentially leading to severe psychological or physical dependence" and require a DEA license for prescription.[28] Because of this potential, writing for the shortest duration possible helps mitigate this risk.

Outside of their use in the setting of malignancy, the risk generally outweighs the benefit of the use of this class with other chronic pain conditions before exhausting other options. Systematic reviews have demonstrated at best small improvements in pain and physical function and high rates of adverse events.[29] In 2016, the US Centers for Disease Control and Prevention released a guideline outlining 12 key points for opioid use in the setting of chronic, nonmalignant pain. The general principles from this guideline are summarized in **Box 2**.[26]

Because of the historical and familiar use of morphine, opioid strength is typically discussed in relation to morphine milligram equivalents (MME), and it is this measure that typically guides escalation and deescalation programs. When initiating opioids, clinicians should start with the lowest effective dose of immediate-release opioids. Escalations should be made slowly in both terms of dosage and the time between increases. Escalation should always be aimed at the lowest effective MME regimen. If a patient has responded to opioid analgesics and is at a stable daily dosage, long-acting opioids with short-acting opioids for breakthrough pain may be considered. To convert to long-acting formulation, convert all current opioid agents to their equianalgesic MME to calculate a total daily dose (**Table 4**).[26] Because of individual differences in metabolism and pharmacodynamics, clinicians typically reduce the total daily dose by 25% to 50% for safety when transitioning between opioids. Divide the desired daily dose by number of doses per day to calculate the MME per dose and convert this to the equianalgesic dose of the selected long-acting opioid. Oral formulations are typically preferred, but transdermal routes may be chosen for individuals with poor gastrointestinal tract absorption, dysphagia, constipation, or those who are unable to tolerate the number of tablets required to manage their symptoms. When

---

**Box 2**
**Summary of recommendations from 2016 Centers for Disease Control and Prevention guideline for prescribing opioids for chronic pain**

- Consider other options before initiating or continuing opioid therapy for chronic nonmalignant pain
- Use shared decision making to establish goals of care and expectations before prescription and continuation
- Use immediate-release opioids as initial therapy and at the lowest effective dosage
- If escalation is necessary, reassess the ongoing need at 50 MME per day. Use caution going over 90 MME per day and consider pain management consultation for dosages over this level
- Use short durations of acute pain prescriptions to help prevent chronic use; 3 days often suffices
- Frequent reevaluation of benefits and harms of therapy should occur with patients at a minimum of 3-month intervals
- Use monitoring of state prescription drug databases and urine drug testing to help curb risk of overdose and/or diversion
- Avoid prescribing opioids and benzodiazepines when possible
- Assist patients to obtain treatment for opioid use disorder if needed

---

deescalating dosages, aim for a 10% reduction per week to help minimize symptoms of withdrawal and achieve success with deescalation.

Opioid use must be continually reassessed for safety and efficacy. Risk mitigation strategies should be used, including informed consent, recurrent evaluations of risk factors for harm, naloxone prescription, and avoidance of concurrent benzodiazepine use.[26] Clinicians must be cognizant of signs of misuse and diversion and ready to provide treatment or referral if opioid use disorder is identified.

## NEUROPATHIC PAIN

Anticonvulsant and antidepressant medications are generally considered first line for neuropathic pain. **Table 5** presents a summary of the magnitude of benefit for medications for the treatment of neuropathic pain, and for fibromyalgia specifically. When comparing anticonvulsants with each other or with SNRIs, there was no significant difference in patient-oriented outcomes.[1] In fibromyalgia, SNRI antidepressants and anticonvulsants show small improvements in pain and function.[1] Memantine can also result in improvements in pain, function, and quality of life compared with placebo.

There is limited evidence for the use of acetaminophen, NSAIDs, or muscle relaxants for this type of pain. Capsaicin 8% patch has demonstrated improvement in postherpetic neuralgia pain,[15] but evidence in other neuropathic pain disorders is lacking.

## COMBINATION REGIMENS

After trialing one class of medications, it may be appropriate to consider combining different classes. Maximizing nonpharmacologic interventions is the best first step, but consideration can be made to any combination of the above medications. Although combination therapy in acute pain conditions has some evidence supporting its use, high-quality data are lacking to support one combination over another in the treatment of chronic pain management.[30] In general, avoid any combinations with

**Table 4**
**Morphine milligram equivalents conversion factors**

| Opioid | MME Conversion Factor |
|---|---|
| Morphine | 1 |
| Codeine | 0.15 |
| Hydrocodone | 1 |
| Oxycodone | 1.5 |
| Fentanyl (µg/h) | 2.4 |
| Oxymorphone | 3 |
| Hydromorphone | 4 |

Commonly available opioids and associated MMEs.
*Adapted from* Dowell D, Haegerich TM, Chou R. CDC Guideline for Prescribing Opioids for Chronic Pain — United States, 2016. MMWR Recomm Rep 2016;65(No. RR-1):1 to 49.

synergistic deleterious side effects (eg, CNS depression). Medication choices should consider comorbid conditions, side-effect profiles, cost, and access. The best successful combination therapy likely includes a multimodal mixture of pharmacologic and nonpharmacologic therapies.

## SPECIAL POPULATIONS

As with the prescription of any therapeutic regimen, certain populations have specific considerations in the pharmacologic management of chronic pain. Renal and hepatic impairment should be considered when selecting medications and dosage. For example, NSAIDs can further diminish kidney function or even precipitate acute kidney injury in geriatric patients and younger patients with other comorbidities.[31] For pregnant patients, work on maximizing nonpharmacologic interventions and use

**Table 5**
**Magnitude of benefit of medications for neuropathic pain**

| Indication | Medication | Short-Term Pain Relief | Short-Term Function Improvement | Short-Term QoL |
|---|---|---|---|---|
| Neuropathic pain | Duloxetine | Small | Small | Small |
| | Pregabalin/gabapentin | Small | None | None |
| | Oxcarbazepine | Small | No evidence | None |
| | Capsaicin patch | None | No evidence | No evidence |
| Fibromyalgia | Duloxetine | Small | Small | Small |
| | Pregabalin/gabapentin | Small | Small | None |
| | Memantine | Moderate | Moderate | Moderate |
| | Cyclobenzaprine | No evidence | No evidence | No evidence |

Magnitude of benefit of selected medications for neuropathic pain and fibromyalgia. Short term is defined as 1 to <6 mo following treatment.
*Abbreviation:* QoL, quality of life.
*Data from* McDonagh MS, Selph SS, Buckley DI et al. Nonopioid Pharmacologic Treatments for Chronic Pain. Comparative Effectiveness Review No. 228. (Prepared by the Pacific Northwest Evidence-based Practice Center under Contract No. 290–2015–00009-I.) AHRQ Publication No. 20-EHC010. Rockville, MD: Agency for Healthcare Research and Quality; April 2020.

**Table 6**
**Considerations for special populations**

| Population | Recommendations |
|---|---|
| Geriatric | • If needed, use the lowest possible dose of NSAIDs<br>• Avoid NSAIDs with longer half-lives to help reduce risk of acute kidney injury or chronic kidney disease<br>• Consider avoiding TCAs (especially the tertiary amines) due to their anticholinergic side effects |
| Pregnancy | • Acetaminophen is first-line agent<br>• Avoid NSAIDs in 3rd trimester<br>• Be cautious with opioid use to avoid the risk of neonatal abstinence syndrome<br>• SNRIs, TCAs, pregabalin, and gabapentin have better safety profiles in pregnancy if pain control required beyond acetaminophen[10] |
| Hepatic impairment | • Avoid acetaminophen-containing compounds in patients with severe liver impairment and severe active liver disease<br>• Dosages up to 2 g/d appear to be safe in patients with cirrhosis and milder forms of hepatic impairment |
| Renal impairment | • Minimize systemic NSAID use in patients with CKD (and even topical NSAIDs in advanced CKD) to avoid disease progression<br>• The anticonvulsants require renal dosage adjustments |

Considerations for pharmacologic pain management for special populations.
*Abbreviation*: CKD, chronic kidney disease.

acetaminophen if pharmacotherapy is necessary.[32] Similarly, most chronic pain medications are discouraged in geriatric patients given the broad side-effect profile.[33] Consider acetaminophen and topical lidocaine patches as the first-line therapy in this population. If geriatric patients require additional pain control, discuss the potential risks and benefits with the patient, begin at the lowest dose and gradually increase as needed, monitor for adverse effects, and frequently reassess to determine if functional and pain management goals are being met. **Table 6** describes some common recommendations for specific populations.

## SUMMARY

There are many available pharmacologic classes used in the treatment of chronic pain, including acetaminophen, oral NSAIDs, topical medications, muscle relaxers, anticonvulsant medications, antidepressants, and opioids. Nonopioid medications result in small to moderate improvements in pain and function with limited differences in efficacy and outcomes between classes and doses of the drugs. Nonopioid medications are preferred to opioid medications in noncancer pain because of the high rates of adverse events as well as the risk of misuse and use disorder. Further research is needed to determine the specific efficacy of each medication for individual pain syndromes. Medications can be used as monotherapy or in combination and can be one component of a multimodal treatment plan. Unfortunately, there are no high-quality studies addressing the efficacy of specific combinations for the management of chronic pain. Pharmacologic management should be tailored based on patient preference, comorbid conditions, side-effect profile, cost, and access. Clinicians should engage their patients in shared decision making to tailor the treatment regimen for the best outcomes of the patient.

## CLINICS CARE POINTS

- Pharmacologic management can be used as a component of a patient-centered multimodal care plan for chronic pain.
- Medication choice should be individualized and consider comorbid conditions, age, reproductive status, adverse effect profiles, cost, and patient values.
- Medications should be used at the lowest effective dose to reduce risk of adverse effects.
- Nonopioid medications result in small to moderate improvement in pain and function.
- Opioid medications should be used with extreme caution and only after shared decision making when safer alternatives have been exhausted.

## DISCLOSURE

The authors have nothing to disclose.

## REFERENCES

1. McDonagh MS, Selph SS, Buckley DI, et al. Nonopioid pharmacologic treatments for chronic pain. Comparative effectiveness review No. 228. Rockville, MD: Agency for Healthcare Research and Quality; 2020. https://doi.org/10.23970/AHRQEPCCER228 (Prepared by the Pacific Northwest Evidence-based Practice Center under Contract No. 290-2015-00009-I.) AHRQ Publication No. 20-EHC010.
2. Wiffen PJ, Knaggs R, Derry S, et al. Paracetamol (acetaminophen) with or without codeine or dihydrocodeine for neuropathic pain in adults. Cochrane Database Syst Rev 2016;12:CD012227.
3. Carville S, Constanti M, Kosky N, et al, Guideline Committee. Chronic pain (primary and secondary) in over 16s: summary of NICE guidance. BMJ 2021;373:n895.
4. Shah NJ, Royer A, John S. Acute liver failure. In: StatPearls [Internet]. Treasure Island (FL): StatPearls Publishing; 2021. Available at: https://www.ncbi.nlm.nih.gov/books/NBK482374/.
5. American Society of Health-System Pharmacists. ISBN-10: 1-58528-654-0, ISBN-13: 978-1-58528-654-6. ISSN: 8756-6028. STAT!Ref Online Electronic Medical Library. In: AHFS drug information® - 2021st. Bethesda, MD: American Society of Health-System Pharmacists®; 2021. Available from: https://online.statref.com/document/cQfe8yqMRNqgSGqm4Qo8Qj. 10/22/2021 12:22:11 PM CDT (UTC -05:00).
6. Bosilkovska M, Walder B, Besson M, et al. Analgesics in patients with hepatic impairment. Drugs 2012;72:1645–69. https://doi.org/10.2165/11635500-000000000-00000.
7. Makris UE, Abrams RC, Gurland B, et al. Management of persistent pain in the older patient: a clinical review. JAMA 2014;312(8):825–36.
8. Enthoven WT, Roelofs PD, Deyo RA, et al. Non-steroidal anti-inflammatory drugs for chronic low back pain. Cochrane Database Syst Rev 2016;2:CD012087. https://doi.org/10.1002/14651858.CD012087.
9. Furst DE. Are there differences among nonsteroidal anti-inflammatory drugs? Comparing acetylated salicylates, nonacetylated salicylates, and nonacetylated nonsteroidal anti-inflammatory drugs. Arthritis Rheum 1994;37:1.

10. Black E, Khor KE, Kennedy D, et al. Medication use and pain management in pregnancy: a critical review. Pain Pract 2019;19(8):875–99.
11. Moore RA, Chi CC, Wiffen PJ, et al. Oral nonsteroidal anti-inflammatory drugs for neuropathic pain. Cochrane Database Syst Rev 2015;10:CD010902.
12. Derry S, Conaghan P, Da Silva JP, et al. Topical NSAIDs for chronic musculoskeletal pain in adults. Cochrane Database Syst Rev 2016;4:CD007400.
13. Murray A. Pharmacist's letter/prescriber's letter. clinical resource, topicals for pain relief. stockton, CA: TRC healthcare. Available at. https://prescriber. therapeuticresearch.com/Content/Segments/PRL/2016/Jan/Topicals-for-Pain-Relief-9274. Accessede.
14. Derry S, Wiffen PJ, Moore RA, et al. Topical lidocaine for neuropathic pain in adults. Cochrane Database Syst Rev 2014;7:CD010958.
15. Derry S, Wiffen PJ, Kalso EA, et al. Topical analgesics for acute and chronic pain in adults - an overview of Cochrane Reviews. Cochrane Database Syst Rev 2017; 12(5):CD008609.
16. Derry S, Rice ASC, Cole P, et al. Topical capsaicin (high concentration) for chronic neuropathic pain in adults. Cochrane Database Syst Rev 2017;1: CD007393.
17. Derry S, Moore RA. Topical capsaicin (low concentration) for chronic neuropathic pain in adults. Cochrane Database Syst Rev 2012;9:CD010111.
18. Tick H, Nielsen A. Academic consortium for integrative medicine & health commentary to Health and Human Services (HHS) on inter-agency task force pain management best practices draft report. Glob Adv Health Med 2019;8. https:// doi.org/10.1177/2164956119857656.
19. Pharmacist's Letter/Prescriber's Letter. Clinical resource, pharmacotherapy of neuropathic pain. Stockton, CA: TRC healthcare. Available at. https:// prescriber.therapeuticresearch.com/Content/Segments/PRL/2015/Nov/ Pharmacotherapy-of-Neuropathic-Pain-9101. Accessed on October 28, 2021.
20. Bonnet U, Scherbaum N. How addictive are gabapentin and pregabalin? A systematic review. Eur Neuropsychopharmacol 2017;27(12):1185–215. https://doi. org/10.1016/j.euroneuro.2017.08.430.
21. United States Food and Drug Administration. FDA warns about serious breathing problems with seizure and nerve pain medicines gabapentin (Neurontin, Gralise, Horizant) and pregabalin (Lyrica, Lyrica CR). 2019. Available at. https://www.fda. gov/drugs/drug-safety-and-availability/fda-warns-about-serious-breathing-problems-seizure-and-nerve-pain-medicines-gabapentin-neurontin.    Accessed October 27, 2021.
22. Pop-Busui R, Boulton AJ, Feldman EL, et al. Diabetic neuropathy: a position statement by the American Diabetes Association. Diabetes Care 2017;40(1): 136–54.
23. Shaheed CA, Maher CG, Williams KA, et al. Efficacy and tolerability of muscle relaxants for low back pain: systematic review and meta-analysis. Eur J Pain 2017; 21:228–37.
24. Chang W. Muscle relaxants for acute and chronic pain. Phys Med Rehabil Clin N Am 2020;31:245–54. https://doi.org/10.1016/j.pmr.2020.01.005. Available at.
25. Chou R, Wagner J, Ahmed AY, et al. Treatments for acute pain: a systematic review. Comparative effectiveness review No. 240. (Prepared by the Pacific Northwest Evidence-based Practice Center under Contract No. 290-2015-00009-I.) AHRQ Publication No. 20(21)-EHC006. Rockville, MD: Agency for Healthcare Research and Quality; 2020. https://doi.org/10.23970/AHRQEPCCER240. Available at.

26. Dowell D, Haegerich TM, Chou R. CDC guideline for prescribing opioids for chronic pain — United States, 2016. MMWR Recomm Rep 2016;65:1–49.
27. The Centers for Disease Control and Prevention. Prescription opioids. 2017. Available at: https://www.cdc.gov/opioids/basics/prescribed.html. Accessed on October 27, 2021.
28. The United States Drug Enforcement Agency. Drug scheduling. Available at: https://www.dea.gov/drug-information/drug-scheduling. Accessed on October 27, 2021.
29. Busse JW, Wang L, Kamaleldin M, et al. Opioids for chronic noncancer pain: a systematic review and meta-analysis. JAMA 2018;320(23):2448–60.
30. Dale R, Stacey B. Multimodal treatment of chronic pain. Med Clin North America 2016;100(1):55–64. https://doi.org/10.1016/j.mcna.2015.08.012.
31. Hörl WH. Nonsteroidal anti-inflammatory drugs and the kidney. Pharmaceuticals (Basel) 2010;3(7):2291–321. https://doi.org/10.3390/ph3072291.
32. Shah S, Banh ET, Koury K, et al. Pain management in pregnancy: multimodal approaches. Pain Res Treat 2015;2015:987483.
33. American Geriatrics Society Beers Criteria Update Expert Panel. Updated AGS beers criteria for potentially inappropriate medication use in older adults. J Am Geriatr Soc 2019;67(4):674–94.
34. Lexicomp online database. UpToDate Inc.. Available at: https://online.lexi.com. Accessed November 1, 2021.

# Nonpharmacologic and Rehabilitative Strategies to Address Chronic Pain

Hiu Ying Joanna Choi, MD

## KEYWORDS

- Nonpharmacologic • Rehabilitation • Exercise • Physical therapy
- Occupational therapy • Aquatic exercise • Multidisciplinary • Education

## KEY POINTS

- Exercise is effective for most chronic pain conditions. Long-term adherence is needed for long-term benefits. Exercise should start at a low intensity and progress in intensity and duration over time.
- Aquatic exercise has similar efficacy to land-based exercises and may be preferred for patients who have difficulty with weight-bearing.
- Weight loss of at least 5% should be recommended in patients with arthritis and high body mass index.
- Patient education and self-management should target fear avoidance, kinesiophobia, pain catastrophizing, and maladaptive behaviors.

## INTRODUCTION

With its benefits and low risk of harm, there has been greater emphasis on nonpharmacologic management of chronic pain. Guidelines recommend nonpharmacological interventions as a core part of treatment in conjunction with other therapies.[1–10] Physical therapy involves exercises and other modalities. Occupational therapy (OT) focuses on optimizing patient's ability to perform daily activities. Aquatic exercises are effective and may be particularly helpful for deconditioned patients. There is limited evidence for taping, orthoses, assistive devices, and thermotherapy. Weight loss is recommended for patients with knee and/or hip arthritis and high body mass index (BMI). Patient education improves self-management and self-efficacy.

Lewis Katz School of Medicine at Temple University, 1316 West Ontario Street, Room 311, Philadelphia, PA 19140, USA
*E-mail address:* hiu.ying.joanna.choi@temple.edu

Prim Care Clin Office Pract 49 (2022) 403–413
https://doi.org/10.1016/j.pop.2022.01.006
0095-4543/22/© 2022 Elsevier Inc. All rights reserved.

primarycare.theclinics.com

## PHYSICAL THERAPY

Physical therapy (PT) is effective and recommended by guidelines as part of comprehensive management of chronic pain conditions.[1-7] Multimodal PT includes therapeutic exercises, manual therapy, electrotherapy, neurodynamic therapy, thermotherapy, and alternative medicine. Effectiveness depends on the modalities used and may or may not be better than exercise alone.[11]

## EXERCISE

Therapeutic exercises are recommended by guidelines as a key component in the management of chronic pain conditions.[1-7] See **Table 1** for a summary of recommendations on therapeutic exercises for chronic pain conditions. Generally, exercise improves physical function and pain.[12] Combination of exercises is generally more effective than one type of exercise alone.[13-16]

Aerobic exercise, exercise performed continuously to increase the cardiac and respiratory rate for a prolonged time, includes running, jogging, walking, cycling, and swimming. Increased blood flow promotes repair and healing.[12,17] It also improves cardiovascular fitness,[13,18] endurance,[13] and physical conditioning.[13] Moderate- to high-intensity aerobic exercise is recommended, except low-impact exercise is preferred in very active disease or severe joint deterioration in rheumatoid arthritis (RA).[17,19]

Strength and resistance exercises involve contracting muscles against resistance (weights, elastic bands, body weight, or water).[12,18] They improve muscle strength and endurance, increasing support of bones and joints.[12] Land-based resistance exercises increase strength more than aquatic resistance exercises.[18] For joint pain, exercises should target weakened muscles surrounding the painful joints.[14,20]

Stretching, flexibility, and range of motion (ROM) exercises involve mobilization of muscles around the targeted joint,[12] to improve muscle stiffness and ROM around the joint.[12,13,18] Alone, ROM exercises have little benefit on pain[18] and are more effective with other exercises or as part of multimodal therapy.[13,16,18,21]

McKenzie method is most commonly used for back pain. Exercises are performed in the direction that causes improvement of symptoms (directional preference), which is manifested by pain becoming more proximal or centralized (centralization). There is limited evidence for its effectiveness on pain and disability,[22] and it is not more effective than other exercises[22,23]

Although evidence exists for the use of exercise therapy in managing chronic pain, there are differences when you look at specific patient-oriented outcomes. Aerobic exercise may be more effective for low back pain, hip and knee osteoarthritis (OA), and fibromyalgia than for RA.[16,17,19,25,31,32] It may be more effective for knee OA versus other types of OA.[16,32] In RA, aerobic exercise and resistance exercise are both effective but are more effective in combination.[13-15] In fibromyalgia, aerobic exercise is more effective than resistance and flexibility exercises.[21,35] In OA[16] and fibromyalgia,[21] ROM exercises may be less effective than aerobic and strengthening exercises and are more effective in combination with other exercises.[16]

Exercises can be supervised in health care settings, individually or in groups, or performed at home. Home exercises may be effective in various chronic pain conditions.[4,19,29,43] However, it is unknown whether it is less effective than supervised exercises.[4,14,15,19,27,29,43]

Exercise programs need to be individually tailored.[5,17,44] Programs that begin at a low intensity and progress gradually in intensity and duration have better adherence and better outcomes.[5,12,18,20,43] Because benefits diminish following cessation of

**Table 1**
**Exercise recommendations for chronic pain conditions**

| Recommendation | Evidence Rating | Comments |
|---|---|---|
| Exercise therapy is recommended for low back pain (with and without radiculopathy),[23–25] osteoarthritis,[26] rheumatoid arthritis (as adjunct to pharmacologic therapy),[19] fibromyalgia,[21,25] shoulder pain,[27,28] and patellofemoral pain syndrome.[29,30] | A | Based on RCTs showing improvement in pain and function |
| Aerobic exercise is recommended for low back pain,[17,31] hip and knee osteoarthritis,[16,32] rheumatoid arthritis,[19] and fibromyalgia.[21,25] | A | Based on RCTs showing improvement in pain and function |
| Strength and resistance exercise is recommended for back pain,[31,33,34] fibromyalgia,[21,35] and rheumatoid arthritis.[19,36] | A | Based on RCTs showing improvement in pain, function, strength, symptom severity, and mental health |
| Strength and resistance exercise may be used for knee osteoarthritis,[16,37,38] hand osteoarthritis,[39] neck pain,[28,40] shoulder pain,[40] and patellofemoral pain syndrome.[41] | B | Based on conflicting or limited evidence from RCTs on pain, function, and disability |
| Stretching, flexibility, and range of motion exercise may be used for osteoarthritis,[16] fibromyalgia,[21,35] back pain,[42] and adhesive capsulitis.[40] | B | Based on limited or conflicting evidence from RCTs showing improvement in pain |

exercise, long-term adherence is required for continued improvement.[1,20,45] Patients need to be counseled that exercise can increase pain at the beginning, but does not accelerate tissue damage,[14,19] and subsides as they gain strength and endurance.[44] Misconceptions about this can cause kinesiophobia, a fear of moving or exercising,[1,43,44] which leads to decreased physical activity.[18]

## OCCUPATIONAL THERAPY

OT aims to optimize patient's ability to perform daily activities.[44,46]

Patient's impairments, activities, and environments are assessed.[47] Body mechanics and maladaptive movements are corrected.[48] Patients are taught how to perform activities safely with positioning strategies and posture correction.[47,49] Activity modifications are planned in advance.[44,47] Energy conservation involves pacing, avoiding repetitive motions, and taking breaks.[9,46] Activity tolerance is improved by techniques to manage pain during daily activities.[44,47]

Joint protection involves education on proper joint mechanics, ergonomic principles, activity modifications, and use of assistive devices; these reduce load and effort during activities, which reduces strain on joints, prevents deformity, but also optimizes functional capacity.[14,46] Patients should be taught to not refrain from using the joint.[10]

Joint protection is effective for improving hand pain in RA[14,43] and OA,[8] especially when combined with ROM and strengthening exercises.[14,15,19,46]

Patients are evaluated for assistive devices and orthoses[46] and their environments for modifications.[46] Ergonomics is used mostly for back and neck pain. Work equipment is adjusted to support the affected joints and reduce strain on muscles.[43]

Workplace interventions may require involving the employer. Patients may need vocational retraining and gradual reintroduction to work duties. Work hours can be reduced or modified, with more frequent breaks or extra time to complete tasks.[5,44,47] Workplace interventions have mixed results on return to work[49] and are not more effective than health care setting–based interventions.[49]

Because of limited evidence for benefit on pain, function, and work productivity, recommendations for OT generally are weak.[5,19,47]

## AQUATIC EXERCISE

Aquatic exercise, performed in a heated pool,[45] may be particularly effective for elderly patients[8] and individuals with deconditioning,[44,49] difficulty with weight bearing,[10,50] or inability to tolerate land-based exercise[1] and can be used as a bridge to land-based exercises.[51] The buoyancy reduces load on joints[50,52] and allows patients to perform movements they are unable to perform on land.[53] Water provides light resistance.[45,52] The warmth improves blood flow,[50] promotes tissue repair[52] and muscle relaxation, and blocks nociceptive signals.[50] Aquatic exercises improve pain, function, and quality of life in OA (especially knee),[1,3,5,6,9,13,16,21,50] fibromyalgia,[18,50] RA,[19] and back pain.[50] There is conflicting evidence whether it is less effective than land-based exercises.[8,20,42,50]

## MULTIDISCIPLINARY REHABILITATION

Multidisciplinary care involves treatment by least 2 disciplines, such as physicians, nurses, PT, OT, social workers, chiropractors, and clinical psychologists.[47] Based on the biopsychosocial model, it usually includes behavioral therapy, medical management (pharmacologic and procedural), exercise, education, and other modalities.[47,54] A common treatment goal and coordination between the disciplines is essential for effective treatment.[44] Sessions can take place in inpatient, outpatient, rehabilitation, community, and workplace settings. There is usually a combination of individual and group therapies.[54] Multidisciplinary care is more effective[49] than medical management and other nonmultidisciplinary interventions alone.[54] Interdisciplinary care involves greater coordination of services with all providers at the same facility[47] and is more effective than less coordinated multidisciplinary programs.[47]

## TAPING, ORTHOSES, AND ASSISTIVE DEVICES

In elastic therapeutic taping, tape is applied to the skin under tension. It is less supportive and restrictive than a brace. Evidence for its effectiveness is generally very low. It has little or no benefit when added to exercise or other interventions.[23,28]

Orthoses prevent movement that aggravate pain and decrease load on the affected joint.[1,20] In general, orthoses have low to very low evidence supporting their use.[20] See **Table 2** for recommendations on taping and orthoses for chronic pain conditions. There is insufficient evidence for lateral wedge insoles for knee OA,[32] knee brace in patellofemoral pain syndrome,[55] lumbar support for back pain,[9,23,56] and wrist/hand[14,15,46,56] and foot orthoses for RA.[56] Modified shoes are not effective for knee or hip OA[4–6,20]

**Table 2**
**Recommendation for taping and orthoses in chronic pain conditions**

| Recommendation | Evidence Rating | Comments |
| --- | --- | --- |
| Taping for knee osteoarthritis (medial taping for lateral compartment osteoarthritis),[59,65,66] plantar fasciitis,[67] shoulder impingement,[40,60] and neck pain.[68] | A | Based on RCTs showing improvement in pain. |
| Taping may be used for back pain.[57,58] | B | Based on conflicting evidence from RCTs on pain and disability. |
| Long-term use of hand orthoses is recommended for hand OA. Short-term use is not recommended.[26,61] | A | Based on meta-analysis of RCTs showing improvement in long-term, but not short-term, pain and function long-term. |
| Functional valgus knee brace is recommended for medial compartment knee OA and is more effective than knee sleeve and lateral wedge insoles.[25,62,63] | A | Based on RCTs and prospective cohort studies showing improvement in pain and function. |
| Foot orthoses may be used for low back pain.[56,69] | B | Based on limited number of RCTs showing improvement in pain and disability. |
| Wrist orthoses may be used for carpal tunnel syndrome.[26,56] | — | Based on conflicting evidence from limited number of RCTs on pain and function. |
| Foot orthoses (insoles) and night splints may be used for plantar fasciitis.[56,59] | B | Based on conflicting evidence from RCTs on improvement in pain and function. |
| Therapy gloves[64] and thumb splints[56] may be used for rheumatoid arthritis. | C | Based on limited and conflicting evidence from RCTs on possible improvement in pain, stiffness. and strength. |

Assistive devices and home adaptations help patients perform daily activities. These include long-handled reachers, sock aids, bath and shower aids, chair and bed raisers, raised toilet seats, perch stools, half steps, grab rails, stair rails, stair lifts, and walk-in showers.[9] Gait assistive devices, including canes, walkers, and crutches, are used commonly in knee and hip OA.[4,9] Although there is insufficient evidence,[3,9,20] most guidelines recommend use of gait aids for hip and/or knee OA.[3–6,8,9] For hand arthritis, use of assistive devices reduces effort and pain during activity.[5,9] Examples include enlarged grips for writing, small nonslip mats for opening objects, electric can openers,[9] leg-adapted knives, and tap turners.[46] There is conflicting evidence on ergonomic keyboards for carpal tunnel syndrome.[70]

## THERMOTHERAPY

Traditionally, ice is used for acute injury and heat for chronic pain.[71] Superficial heat includes hot water bottles, heated stones, heated packs, hot towels, hot baths, steam, heat wraps, heat pads, and infrared heat lamps.[72] Heat increases the pain threshold in free nerve endings and reduces muscle spasm.[73] Cold therapy includes local and whole-body cryotherapy, cold compresses and towels, vapocoolant sprays, ice packs, ice massage, and whole-body ice baths.[72,73] It decreases pain and inflammation by constricting blood flow in muscles and joints and slowing nerve conduction.[53,71–73] When applied for too long, cold therapy can be painful and proinflammatory.[71] Ice should not be in direct contact with the skin and should be applied for no longer than 20 to 30 minutes.[71]

Because of heterogeneity,[4] there is little evidence for their efficacy.[71] Duration of effect is short.[4,70] Guidelines have weak recommendations for thermotherapy as adjunctive therapy for hip, knee, and hand OA.[4,8,9] Cold therapy may be effective for knee arthritis,[10,11,53,71,72] rheumatoid arthritis,[71] and back pain.[72] Heat therapy may be effective for hand OA,[15] back pain,[72] and wrist pain[70] but is not effective for knee arthritis.[11]

## LIFESTYLE

Physical activity is recommended for all adults.[8] Inactivity contributes to deconditioning and decreased strength.[51]

High BMI is associated with progression of hip and knee OA and decreased function and mobility.[5,20,74] Guidelines recommend weight loss for patients with knee with or without hip arthritis who are overweight or obese.[1,3,4,9,20] Weight loss of 5% to 10% improves pain, function, disability, stiffness, quality of life, and depressive symptoms.[4,6,10,11,20,74]

Weight loss interventions are effective for weight loss[75,76]; they may include diet, exercise, and a behavioral component. Effective interventions have regular weight recording and follow-up, explicit weight loss goals, reduced caloric intake, increased fruit and vegetable intake, exercise plans, counseling on healthy eating habits, self-monitoring, coping strategies, and behavioral modifications.[5,11] Diet, including low-calorie diets, alone is effective for weight loss[11,32] but is more effective in combination with exercise for weight loss[74] and pain-related outcomes.[32]

## PATIENT EDUCATION AND SELF-MANAGEMENT

Patient education is recommended as part of multicomponent management of chronic pain.[3,5,9,10,13,42] Education can be given in various formats by a variety of providers.[5] Patients should be educated on their condition, its symptoms and progression,[3,42,77] nature of chronic pain,[77] expectations of treatment,[13] efficacy of nonpharmacologic care,[13] and the unnecessity of imaging and surgery.[11] Unhelpful pain-related beliefs, fear avoidance, kinesiophobia, pain catastrophizing, and maladaptive behaviors should be addressed.[20,77] Education improves psychosocial outcomes, including self-management, knowledge of pain, kinesiophobia, adherence, exercise behavior, coping, pain catastrophizing, and self-efficacy.[3,11,42,77] However, evidence is conflicting for pain, function, and disability.[3,5,9,10,13,19,20,43]

Self-management interventions include education on management of symptoms, self-efficacy building, self-monitoring, self-regulation, pain coping, pain acceptance, barrier identification, problem solving, goal setting, resource utilization, and forming partnerships with health care providers[3,5,42]; they often include education, exercise, and behavioral and lifestyle components.[48]

Both increase self-efficacy (ability to manage one's condition),[48] which is associated with improvements in disability, pain, physical functioning, adherence to physical activity, and health-related quality of life.[48] Both have insufficient evidence as standalone interventions and are recommended as part of comprehensive treatment.[42,48]

## BARRIERS

Nonpharmacological interventions for chronic pain are often underused.[11] Patients are often not aware of nonpharmacological options.[77] Providers often offer it late in care, have a lack of training, and are uncertain about making specific recommendations.[1,77] Other barriers include low self-efficacy, behavioral factors, time, and cost.[1,11,53]

## SUMMARY

Further research is needed to determine which types, intensity, frequency, and duration of exercises are more effective for each condition. There is limited evidence for commonly used long-standing interventions, including OT, aquatherapy, thermotherapy, orthoses, and assistive devices, which would benefit from further research. There should also be further research on newer modalities. With advancement and increasing use of technology in health care, some interventions, such as self-management, education, and exercise, are being delivered remotely. The effectiveness of remotely delivered interventions also requires more research.

## CLINICS CARE POINTS

- Exercise is effective for chronic pain conditions. It should start at a low intensity and progress in intensity and duration over time. Long-term adherence is needed for long-term benefit.
- Aquatic exercise has similar efficacy to land-based exercises and may be preferred for patients who have difficulty with weight-bearing.
- Multidisciplinary and interdisciplinary care are more effective than individual modalities.
- Weight loss of at least 5% should be recommended in patients with arthritis who are overweight or obese.
- Patient education and self-management should target fear avoidance, kinesiophobia, pain catastrophizing, and maladaptive behaviors.

## DISCLOSURE

The author has nothing to disclose.

## REFERENCES

1. Goodman F, Kaiser L, Kelley C, et al. VA/DoD clinical practice guideline for the non-surgical management of hip and knee osteoarthritis. Washington, DC: Department of Veterans Affairs, Department of Defense; 2020. Available at: https://www.healthquality.va.gov/guidelines/cd/oa/index.asp.
2. Qaseem A, Wilt TJ, McLean RM, et al. Clinical Guidelines Committee of the American College of Physicians. Noninvasive Treatments for Acute, Subacute, and Chronic Low Back Pain: a Clinical Practice Guideline From the American College of Physicians. Ann Intern Med 2017;166(7):514–30.
3. Bannuru RR, Osani MC, Vaysbrot EE, et al. OARSI guidelines for the non-surgical management of knee, hip, and polyarticular osteoarthritis. Osteoarthritis Cartilage 2019;27(11):1578–89.

4. Kolasinski SL, Neogi T, Hochberg MC, et al. 2019 American College of Rheumatology/Arthritis Foundation Guideline for the Management of Osteoarthritis of the Hand, Hip, and Knee. Arthritis Care Res (Hoboken) 2020;72(2):149–62.

5. Fernandes L, Hagen KB, Bijlsma JW, et al. European league against rheumatism (EULAR). EULAR recommendations for the non-pharmacological core management of hip and knee osteoarthritis. Ann Rheum Dis 2013;72(7):1125–35.

6. McAlindon TE, Bannuru RR, Sullivan MC, et al. OARSI guidelines for the non-surgical management of knee osteoarthritis. Osteoarthritis Cartilage 2014;22(3):363–88.

7. Macfarlane GJ, Kronisch C, Dean LE, et al. EULAR revised recommendations for the management of fibromyalgia. Ann Rheum Dis 2017;76(2):318–28.

8. Rillo O, Riera H, Acosta C, et al. PANLAR Consensus Recommendations for the Management in Osteoarthritis of Hand, Hip, and Knee. J Clin Rheumatol 2016;22(7):345–54.

9. National Clinical Guideline Centre (UK). Osteoarthritis: care and management in adults. London (United Kingdom): National Institute for Health and Care Excellence; 2014.

10. Kloppenburg M, Kroon FP, Blanco FJ, et al. 2018 update of the EULAR recommendations for the management of hand osteoarthritis. Ann Rheum Dis 2019;78(1):16–24.

11. Dantas LO, Salvini TF, McAlindon TE. Knee osteoarthritis: key treatments and implications for physical therapy. Braz J Phys Ther 2021;25(2):135–46.

12. Geneen LJ, Moore RA, Clarke C, et al. Physical activity and exercise for chronic pain in adults: an overview of Cochrane Reviews. Cochrane Database Syst Rev 2017;4(4):CD011279.

13. Cunningham NR, Kashikar-Zuck S. Nonpharmacological treatment of pain in rheumatic diseases and other musculoskeletal pain conditions. Curr Rheumatol Rep 2013;15(2):306.

14. Ekelman BA, Hooker L, Davis A, et al. Occupational therapy interventions for adults with rheumatoid arthritis: an appraisal of the evidence. Occup Ther Health Care 2014;28(4):347–61.

15. Martin A, Chopra R, Nicassio PM. Nonpharmacologic pain management in inflammatory arthritis. Rheum Dis Clin North Am 2021;47(2):277–95.

16. Uthman OA, van der Windt DA, Jordan JL, et al. Exercise for lower limb osteoarthritis: systematic review incorporating trial sequential analysis and network meta-analysis. BMJ 2013;347:f5555.

17. Gordon R, Bloxham S. A systematic review of the effects of exercise and physical activity on non-specific chronic low back pain. Healthcare (Basel) 2016;4(2):22.

18. Ambrose KR, Golightly YM. Physical exercise as non-pharmacological treatment of chronic pain: Why and when. Best Pract Res Clin Rheumatol 2015;29(1):120–30.

19. Siegel P, Tencza M, Apodaca B, et al. Effectiveness of occupational therapy interventions for adults with rheumatoid arthritis: a systematic review. Am J Occup Ther 2017;71(1). 7101180050p1-7101180050p11.

20. Rice D, McNair P, Huysmans E, et al. Best evidence rehabilitation for chronic pain part 5: osteoarthritis. J Clin Med 2019;8(11):1769.

21. Poole JL, Siegel P. Effectiveness of occupational therapy interventions for adults with fibromyalgia: a systematic review. Am J Occup Ther 2017;71(1). 7101180040p1-7101180040p10.

22. Lam OT, Strenger DM, Chan-Fee M, et al. Effectiveness of the McKenzie method of mechanical diagnosis and therapy for treating low back pain: literature review with meta-analysis. J Orthop Sports Phys Ther 2018;48(6):476–90.

23. Chou R, Deyo R, Friedly J, et al. Noninvasive treatments for low back pain. Rockville (MD): Agency for Healthcare Research and Quality (US); 2016. Report No.: 16-EHC004-EF.

24. Chou R, Deyo R, Friedly J, et al. Nonpharmacologic therapies for low back pain: a systematic review for an American College of Physicians Clinical Practice Guideline. Ann Intern Med 2017;166(7):493–505.

25. Skelly AC, Chou R, Dettori JR, et al. Noninvasive nonpharmacological treatment for chronic pain: a systematic review update. Rockville (MD): Agency for Healthcare Research and Quality (US); 2020. Report No.: 20-EHC009.

26. Peprah K, MacDougall D. Orthotic bracing or splinting of upper extremities in patients with chronic, non-cancer pain: a review of clinical effectiveness. Ottawa (ON): Canadian Agency for Drugs and Technologies in Health; 2020.

27. Littlewood C, Malliaras P, Chance-Larsen K. Therapeutic exercise for rotator cuff tendinopathy: a systematic review of contextual factors and prescription parameters. Int J Rehabil Res 2015;38(2):95–106.

28. Gross A, Kay TM, Paquin JP, et al. Cervical Overview Group. Exercises FOR mechanical neck disorders. Cochrane Database Syst Rev 2015;1:CD004250.

29. van der Heijden RA, Lankhorst NE, van Linschoten R, et al. Exercise for treating patellofemoral pain syndrome. Cochrane Database Syst Rev 2015;1:CD010387.

30. Alba-Martín P, Gallego-Izquierdo T, Plaza-Manzano G, et al. Effectiveness of therapeutic physical exercise in the treatment of patellofemoral pain syndrome: a systematic review. J Phys Ther Sci 2015;27(7):2387–90.

31. Owen PJ, Miller CT, Mundell NL, et al. Which specific modes of exercise training are most effective for treating low back pain? Network meta-analysis. Br J Sports Med 2020;54(21):1279–87.

32. Katz JN, Arant KR, Loeser RF. Diagnosis and treatment of hip and knee osteoarthritis: a review. JAMA 2021;325(6):568–78.

33. Vadalà G, Russo F, De Salvatore S, et al. Physical activity for the treatment of chronic low back pain in elderly patients: a systematic review. J Clin Med 2020;9(4):1023.

34. Wewege MA, Booth J, Parmenter BJ. Aerobic vs. resistance exercise for chronic non-specific low back pain: A systematic review and meta-analysis. J Back Musculoskelet Rehabil 2018;31(5):889–99.

35. Sosa-Reina MD, Nunez-Nagy S, Gallego-Izquierdo T, et al. Effectiveness of Therapeutic Exercise in Fibromyalgia Syndrome: A Systematic Review and Meta-Analysis of Randomized Clinical Trials. Biomed Res Int 2017;2017:2356346.

36. Baillet A, Vaillant M, Guinot M, et al. Efficacy of resistance exercises in rheumatoid arthritis: meta-analysis of randomized controlled trials. Rheumatology (Oxford) 2012;51(3):519.

37. Newberry SJ, FitzGerald J, SooHoo NF, et al. Treatment of osteoarthritis of the knee: an update review. Rockville (MD): Agency for Healthcare Research and Quality (US); 2017. Report No.: 17-EHC011-EF.

38. Bartholdy C, Juhl C, Christensen R, et al. The role of muscle strengthening in exercise therapy for knee osteoarthritis: A systematic review and meta-regression analysis of randomized trials. Semin Arthritis Rheum 2017;47(1):9–21.

39. Magni NE, McNair PJ, Rice DA. The effects of resistance training on muscle strength, joint pain, and hand function in individuals with hand osteoarthritis: a systematic review and meta-analysis. Arthritis Res Ther 2017;19(1):131.

40. Marik TL, Roll SC. Effectiveness of occupational therapy interventions for musculoskeletal shoulder conditions: a systematic review. Am J Occup Ther 2017;71(1). 7101180020p1-7101180020p11.
41. Saltychev M, Dutton RA, Laimi K, et al. Effectiveness of conservative treatment for patellofemoral pain syndrome: A systematic review and meta-analysis. J Rehabil Med 2018;50(5):393–401.
42. Delitto A, George SZ, Van Dillen L, et al. Orthopaedic Section of the American Physical Therapy Association. Low back pain. J Orthop Sports Phys Ther 2012; 42(4):A1–57.
43. Grazio S, Grubišić F, Brnić V. Rehabilitation of patients with spondyloarthritis: a narrative review. Med Glas (Zenica) 2019;16(2).
44. Mathews M, Davin S. Chronic pain rehabilitation. Neurosurg Clin N Am 2014; 25(4):799–802.
45. Dadabo J, Fram J, Jayabalan P. Noninterventional therapies for the management of knee osteoarthritis. J Knee Surg 2019;32(1):46–54.
46. Hammond A. What is the role of the occupational therapist? Best Pract Res Clin Rheumatol 2004;18(4):491–505.
47. Hylands-White N, Duarte RV, Raphael JH. An overview of treatment approaches for chronic pain management. Rheumatol Int 2017;37(1):29–42.
48. Bonakdar RA. Integrative pain management. Med Clin North Am 2017;101(5): 987–1004.
49. Wegrzynek PA, Wainwright E, Ravalier J. Return to work interventions for chronic pain: a systematic review. Occup Med (Lond) 2020;70(4):268–77.
50. Verhagen AP, Cardoso JR, Bierma-Zeinstra SM. Aquatic exercise & balneotherapy in musculoskeletal conditions. Best Pract Res Clin Rheumatol 2012;26(3): 335–43.
51. Esser S, Bailey A. Effects of exercise and physical activity on knee osteoarthritis. Curr Pain Headache Rep 2011;15(6):423–30.
52. Corvillo I, Armijo F, Álvarez-Badillo A, et al. Efficacy of aquatic therapy for neck pain: a systematic review. Int J Biometeorol 2020;64(6):915–25.
53. Thomas DA, Maslin B, Legler A, et al. Role of alternative therapies for chronic pain syndromes. Curr Pain Headache Rep 2016;20(5):29.
54. Scascighini L, Sprott H. Chronic nonmalignant pain: a challenge for patients and clinicians. Nat Clin Pract Rheumatol 2008;4(2):74–81.
55. Smith TO, Drew BT, Meek TH, et al. Knee orthoses for treating patellofemoral pain syndrome. Cochrane Database Syst Rev 2015;2015(12):CD010513.
56. Healy A, Farmer S, Pandyan A, et al. A systematic review of randomised controlled trials assessing effectiveness of prosthetic and orthotic interventions. PLoS One 2018;13(3):e0192094.
57. Li Y, Yin Y, Jia G, et al. Effects of kinesiotape on pain and disability in individuals with chronic low back pain: a systematic review and meta-analysis of randomized controlled trials. Clin Rehabil 2019;33(4):596–606.
58. Luz Júnior MAD, Almeida MO, Santos RS, et al. Effectiveness of kinesio taping in patients with chronic nonspecific low back pain: a systematic review with meta-analysis. Spine (Phila Pa 1976) 2019;44(1):68–78.
59. Schuitema D, Greve C, Postema K, et al. Effectiveness of mechanical treatment for plantar fasciitis: a systematic review. J Sport Rehabil 2019;29(5):657–74.
60. Taylor RL, O'Brien L, Brown T. A scoping review of the use of elastic therapeutic tape for neck or upper extremity conditions. J Hand Ther 2014;27(3):235–45 [quiz: 246].

61. Spaans AJ, van Minnen LP, Kon M, et al. Conservative treatment of thumb base osteoarthritis: a systematic review. J Hand Surg Am 2015;40(1):16–21.e1-6.
62. Gohal C, Shanmugaraj A, Tate P, et al. Effectiveness of valgus offloading knee braces in the treatment of medial compartment knee osteoarthritis: a systematic review. Sports Health 2018;10(6):500–14.
63. Cudejko T, van der Esch M, van der Leeden M, et al. Effect of soft braces on pain and physical function in patients with knee osteoarthritis: systematic review with meta-analyses. Arch Phys Med Rehabil 2018;99(1):153–63.
64. Hammond A, Jones V, Prior Y. The effects of compression gloves on hand symptoms and hand function in rheumatoid arthritis and hand osteoarthritis: a systematic review. Clin Rehabil 2016;30(3):213–24.
65. Ramírez-Vélez R, Hormazábal-Aguayo I, Izquierdo M, et al. Effects of kinesio taping alone versus sham taping in individuals with musculoskeletal conditions after intervention for at least one week: a systematic review and meta-analysis. Physiotherapy 2019;105(4):412–20.
66. Ouyang JH, Chang KH, Hsu WY, et al. Non-elastic taping, but not elastic taping, provides benefits for patients with knee osteoarthritis: systemic review and meta-analysis. Clin Rehabil 2018;32(1):3–17.
67. Luo WH, Li Y. Current evidence does support the use of KT to treat chronic knee pain in short term: a systematic review and meta-analysis. Pain Res Manag 2021; 2021:5516389.
68. Vanti C, Bertozzi L, Gardenghi I, et al. Effect of taping on spinal pain and disability: systematic review and meta-analysis of randomized trials. Phys Ther 2015;95(4):493–506.
69. Kong L, Zhou X, Huang Q, et al. The effects of shoes and insoles for low back pain: a systematic review and meta-analysis of randomized controlled trials. Res Sports Med 2020;28(4):572–87.
70. Huisstede BM, Hoogvliet P, Randsdorp MS, et al. Carpal tunnel syndrome. Part I: effectiveness of nonsurgical treatments–a systematic review. Arch Phys Med Rehabil 2010;91(7):981–1004.
71. Guillot X, Tordi N, Mourot L, et al. Cryotherapy in inflammatory rheumatic diseases: a systematic review. Expert Rev Clin Immunol 2014;10(2):281–94.
72. French SD, Cameron M, Walker BF, et al. Superficial heat or cold for low back pain. Cochrane Database Syst Rev 2006;(1):CD004750.
73. Glversen MD. Rehabilitation interventions for pain and disability in osteoarthritis: a review of interventions including exercise, manual techniques, and assistive devices. Orthop Nurs 2012;31(2):103–8.
74. Vincent HK, Heywood K, Connelly J, et al. Obesity and weight loss in the treatment and prevention of osteoarthritis. PM R 2012;4(5 Suppl):S59–67.
75. Cooper L, Ryan CG, Ells LJ, et al. Weight loss interventions for adults with overweight/obesity and chronic musculoskeletal pain: a mixed methods systematic review. Obes Rev 2018;19(7):989–1007.
76. Robins H, Perron V, Heathcote LC, et al. Pain neuroscience education: state of the art and application in pediatrics. Children (Basel) 2016;3(4):43.
77. George SZ, Lentz TA, Goertz CM. Back and neck pain: in support of routine delivery of non-pharmacologic treatments as a way to improve individual and population health. Transl Res 2021;234:129–40.

# Trauma and Behavioral Health Care for Patients with Chronic Pain

Daniel Salahuddin, MD, MPH[a],*,[1], Tracey Conti, MD[b]

## KEYWORDS

• Trauma • PTSD • Chronic pain • Integrated care

## KEY POINTS

• The cause of pain is multifactorial and must be understood through a multidimensional lens.
• There is a strong relationship between chronic pain and mental illness, specifically post-traumatic stress disorder.
• It is important for primary care providers to be acquainted with the various strategies and modalities for addressing pain. These interventions must be tailored to the individual and their circumstance.

## INTRODUCTION

Pain is defined by the International Association for the Study of Pain as an unpleasant sensory and emotional experience associated with actual or potential tissue damage or described in terms of such damage and is deemed chronic if it persists for 3 months or longer, persisting beyond the healing of the initial injury or disease process.[1] Consequently, pain has been traditionally conceptualized as being directly associated with the extent of physical pathology that may be present; however, significant variation in how patients report pain in relation to the presence or absence of physical pathology and low association between impairments and disability indicate that factors other than physical pathology contribute to reports of pain.[2] Thus pain may be better understood as a multidimensional, complex, subjective, perceptual phenomenon.[3] This phenomenon can be further broken down into different components, including sensory, cognitive, behavioral, and emotional.[4] This article reviews the interplay between

[a] Department of Psychiatry, University of Pittsburgh Medical Center, 3811 O'Hara Street, Pittsburgh, PA 15213, USA; [b] Department of Family Medicine, University of Pittsburgh School of Medicine, 4420 Bayard Street, Suite 520, Pittsburgh, PA 15213, USA
[1] 4420 Bayard Street, Suite 520, Pittsburgh, PA 15213
* Corresponding author.
E-mail address: salahuddindr@upmc.edu
Twitter: @DanDouyonMD (D.S.); @TraceyConti2 (T.C.)

Prim Care Clin Office Pract 49 (2022) 415–423
https://doi.org/10.1016/j.pop.2022.04.001
0095-4543/22/© 2022 Elsevier Inc. All rights reserved.

pain and mental illness, with a specific focus on posttraumatic stress disorder (PTSD), psychological factors that influence pain, and various modalities that have been studied and implemented to address chronic pain and comorbid PTSD.

## CHRONIC PAIN AND PSYCHIATRY

Chronic pain is a public health problem that affects approximately 100 million people in the United States.[5] It can be caused by a variety of factors including natural degenerative changes that may occur in the body, disease conditions, or physical injury. In addition, chronic pain can develop secondary to traumatic events, such as work-related injuries, motor-vehicle accidents, or injuries associated with engagement in military combat.[3,5] As chronicity of the pain increases, emotional distress, functional limitations, and increased utilization of the health care system tend to occur, creating a cycle that is self-perpetuating and self-reinforcing.[3]

Among those affected by chronic pain, patients with comorbid mental illness are overrepresented.[6] Psychiatric disorders are commonly associated with alterations in pain processing, whereas chronic pain may impair emotional and neurocognitive functioning. There are many theories as to why patients with psychiatric illness are over-represented among patients with chronic pain, and thus elucidating the mechanisms underlying the connection between these 2 entities has been an area of active investigation. There is thought to be neurobiological overlap between the processing of pain and stress, reward, and motivational regulation, which may be relevant to psychiatric morbidity.[6] More specifically, sensory areas of the brain are recruited by both acute and chronic pain; however, the latter uses a more complex phenomenon that engages a wider stress-related neural network with emotional, motivational, and cognitive components that converge on the mesocorticolimbic dopaminergic and endogenous opioid circuits, which are involved in reward/salience/motivational mechanisms. Thus, the neuroanatomical and functional overlap between pain and emotion/reward/motivation brain circuitry suggests integration and mutual modulation of these systems.[6]

## CHRONIC PAIN AND POSTTRAUMATIC STRESS DISORDER

PTSD is defined by the revised fifth edition of the Diagnostic and Statistical Manual of Mental Health Disorders[7] as a psychiatric disorder that may occur at least 1 month after witnessing or experiencing a life-threatening event such as combat, disaster, assault/violence, or an automobile accident. Symptoms include intrusive distressing memories or recurrent distressing dreams, persistent avoidance of stimuli associated with the traumatic event, negative alterations in cognitions and mood associated with the traumatic event, marked alteration in arousal and reactivity associated with the traumatic event, and these disturbances causing significant distress or impairment in social, occupational, or other important areas of functioning.[7] PTSD has a lifetime incidence of 7% but can range from 20% to 50% in high-risk groups, including victims of motor vehicle accidents, sexual assault, and persons with military combat exposure.[8] The rate of PTSD is much higher among people with chronic pain, and individuals with these comorbidities report greater PTSD symptoms, pain, anxiety, depression, disability, and opioid use than those with only one of these conditions.[4,5,9] Studies have noted the presence of PTSD in 10% to 50% of chronic pain cases, compared with 6% of men and 12% of women in the general population.[4,5,10,11] A recent meta-analysis found variations in the prevalence of PTSD depending on chronic pain types/subgroups of patients with chronic pain, with 50% of veterans with chronic pain having comorbid PTSD.[10] The study also found that all subgroups of chronic pain type had higher comorbid PTSD than the general population.[10] Furthermore, among patients with chronic pain in a nationally representative sample, the prevalence of opioid use disorder (OUD) was higher among those with PTSD than those without PTSD.[12] The investigators also found that musculoskeletal (MSK) and nerve pain conditions are associated with increased odds of OUD but that only MSK pain conditions display an additive relationship on OUD when combined with PTSD.[12] A 2015 study of chronic back pain showed that patients with lower back pain and trauma exposure had more generalized hyperalgesia with lower thresholds in both painful and nonpainful areas, whereas patients with low back pain without a previous trauma history demonstrated more localized hyperalgesia with decreased thresholds only in the pain-affected area of the back.[8] These findings suggest an augmented central pain processing in patients with both chronic pain and trauma, whereas patients with only chronic pain and no trauma show only local changes (alterations only in the painful area), suggesting regional sensitization processes.[8] A 2017 study among unhoused persons with mental illness revealed that 43% reported moderate-to-severe chronic pain and that mental illness was an independent predictor of chronic pain.[13] Among participants with PTSD, 52% reported chronic pain.[13]

Given the bidirectional association and both symptomatic and conceptual overlap between chronic pain and PTSD, several frameworks have been proposed that help explain the reinforced relationship. Among the most prominent is the fear-avoidant cycle, also referred to as the "mutual maintenance" cycle of chronic pain and PTSD. Fear-avoidance cycles associated with both chronic pain and PTSD are self-perpetuating, resting on a common foundation of avoidance that precludes recovery and reinforces maladaptive beliefs, ineffective behaviors, distressing symptoms, and functional limitations.[3] As a result, this cycle may influence the development of each condition over time, may serve to maintain them, and may interact in ways that affect the outcome of either condition[3]; this is to say that a feared stimuli such as pain, paired with emotional trauma and its recollections, can become a conditioned stimulus evoking fear and anxiety responses that in turn augment subjective pain perception and its neural correlates, leading to additional deterioration and avoidance of pain- and trauma-related situations.[3–6,14] Therefore, these patients are at high risk to be controlled by pain and/or distressing symptoms.

From the neurobiological perspective, increased central opioidergic tone along with robust elevations in endogenous opioid concentrations in the cerebral spinal fluid and plasma are relatively consistent clinical findings in PTSD. Therefore, similar to long-term users of opioid analgesics, exaggerated central nervous system opioidergic activity in PTSD could contribute to the sensitized pain phenomenon potentially mediated via amplification of the excitatory (glutamatergic) neurotransmission.[6] The hypothalamus-pituitary-adrenal axis has also been implicated as a mediating neurobiological pathway between chronic pain and chronic stress; however, this is still under investigation.[15] The investigators note that unifying the processes of chronic pain and chronic stress under one theoretic framework would be enhanced by understanding how different chronic painful or stressful conditions induce continuous emotional learning, centered particularly around the properties and remodeling of amygdala and hippocampus.[15]

## TREATMENT GOALS FOR COMORBID CHRONIC PAIN AND POSTTRAUMATIC STRESS DISORDER

Treatment goals for patients with both chronic pain and PTSD should focus on improvement in daily functioning and increasing quality of life by deflecting or minimizing the shared role of fear avoidance.[3] Bosco and colleagues propose integrated care treatment components that can achieve these goals through various means. These components include the following: psychoeducation to better understand the interaction between the behaviors, emotions, and cognitions that reflect the development of ascribing meaning, or appraisals, related to both chronic pain and PTSD; reducing chronic pain and PTSD-related avoidance behaviors by the systemic practice of increasingly challenging avoided stimuli; initiating interventions to reduce depression, such as facilitating reengagement in previously enjoyed activities; cognitive restructuring, either through thought logs with associated exercises to challenge maladaptive automatic thoughts or indirectly through the process of strengthening esteem and sense of agency/efficacy and worth via behavioral assignments and habituation; addressing and correcting attentional biases that develop in response to both chronic pain and PTSD; normalizing emotional responses and contributing physiologic sensations, including ongoing identification and confrontation of avoidance or escape behaviors; and lastly incorporating structured relaxation as a means to reduce tension and help regulate physiologic symptoms of anxiety.[3]

When assessing treatment efficacy in this setting, outcome measures that assess chronic pain, PTSD, cognitive functioning, coping behaviors, and specific functional domains are necessary to assess and track current functioning and levels of distress in those with chronic pain and PTSD to identify their emotional and behavioral sequelae and to assess their response to concurrent treatment.[3] These complex and multifactorial processes emphasize the importance of integrated care in the management of this patient population.

## PSYCHOLOGICAL FACTORS INFLUENCING PAIN

Before exploring the various therapeutic modalities for chronic pain and PTSD, it is important to understand the psychological factors that influence the experience of pain, as well as the overall effects of pain on both psychological functioning and day-to-day functioning.[16] Gaining a better understanding of this perspective may help health care providers to better empathize, connect with, and validate patients who are suffering from chronic pain, which in turn can help to strengthen the therapeutic alliance.

The psychological factors that influence pain are grouped into 3 categories: catastrophizing, pain beliefs, and pain coping response.[16] The remainder of this section further explores these factors.

Catastrophizing involves ruminating about devastating thoughts regarding pain and the role it plays in a patient's life. Expressed sentiments may include "I'm never going to get over this pain" and "I can't stop thinking about the pain." It is the strongest and most consistent predictor of patient pain and suffering of all the psychosocial factors.[16] In addition, patients who catastrophize report higher levels of pain, depression, anxiety, distress, and disability compared with patients who do not catastrophize.[16] Research shows that reducing or stopping catastrophizing results in improvements on many outcome variables, including pain intensity, psychological functioning, and activity level. In addition, lower levels of catastrophizing are associated with maintaining treatment gains made in both psychological and physical functioning.[16] Thus, it is critical for providers to assess for and address catastrophizing with patients when it is present.

Pain beliefs are the meanings that patients ascribe to their pain.[16] These beliefs are composed of 4 domains: control and self-efficacy (the belief that patients can control their pain experience), pain acceptance (the belief of accepting suffering and pain as components of a rich experience, which in turn helps patients become more open to other emotional experiences, such as joy and a sense of meaning), disability (the belief that one is disabled by pain and lives their life accordingly at the expense of living a more active life), harm (the belief that pain is a sign of physical damage and that activities resulting in more pain should be avoided), pain management responsibility (the belief in a purely biomedical model of suffering, where pain is a sign of peripheral damage and that this damage has to heal), analgesic medication use (the belief about the appropriateness of analgesic medication for chronic pain, usually in favor), and lastly solicitude (belief that other people, notably family, should be attentive when the patient is experiencing pain).[16]

Although pain-related catastrophizing and pain beliefs reflect a patient's thought process and understanding of their pain, pain coping reflects what patients do to manage pain and its broad effects.[16] There are 8 coping domains most relevant to patient functioning, 5 adaptive and 3 maladaptive. The adaptive domains include coping self-statements, which are calming and reassuring thoughts in response to pain and can be thought of as the opposite of catastrophizing. It should be noted that catastrophizing is more strongly negatively associated with functioning than coping self-statements are associated positively with functioning; therefore, it may be more important to discourage catastrophizing than it is to encourage coping self-statements; however, each have a role regarding promoting patient function. Pacing is an adaptive domain that reflects how one goes about controlling the rate or speed at which one performs tasks; this allows patients to maintain an appropriate level of activity, thereby achieving their most valued goals and meet their most valued responsibilities. Because the objective of pacing is to achieve important goals, rest in response to pain is not considered to be adequately pacing because the choice to rest is being predicated on pain rather than on their goals. The opposite phenomenon can also occur in which patients base what they do on their level of pain, or pain relief, rather than on their most valued goals. Thus, the appropriate strategy for pacing is to determine the appropriate level of activity required to achieve goals and live one's life and stick with the level of activity, assuming that it is reasonable, as opposed to centering around the presence or absence of pain.[16] Task persistence is the continuation of normal (reasonable) activity despite pain and is central to adaptive pain management if physically safe. Exercise and stretching is an adaptive domain that should be used regularly, given the fact that individuals with chronic pain are at risk for muscle and tendon atrophy, particularly in areas of the body where they hurt the most.[16] Of note, providers should work alongside their patients to identify exercises that are safe, especially if there are other comorbidities present. The last of the adaptive domains include seeking social support, which emphasizes ongoing and non–pain-contingent affection and emotional support.[16]

Maladaptive coping domains include guarding, which keeps the body stiff or still or limits the use of a body part. It is initially adaptive to facilitate healing during early phase of injury; however, guarding that extends beyond healing time is thought to produce (rather than inhibit) physical disability and greater pain and can also cause muscles and tendons to weaken over time, increasing the likelihood of spasms and paradoxically increasing pain.[16] Resting can be effective if used wisely to maximize activity and energy, as described in pacing; however, some patients rest far too much when experiencing pain, which ultimately leads to muscle and tendon weakness and limits opportunities to engage in valued activities. Consequently, patients should be discouraged to rest when they hurt and encouraged to rest as a reinforcement for engaging in an important activity.[16] Lastly, asking for help can be maladaptive if support is given in a pain-contingent context. This pattern has been consistently shown to predict poorer patient functioning, may undermine patient confidence, and can turn someone who might otherwise be able to increase their strength, endurance, and engagement in life, into a disabled and demoralized individual. An example of how to discuss this with a patient would be to avoid asking for assistance with chores or tasks they are able to complete, even when they feel pain.[16]

Although the aforementioned psychological factors provide a framework for conceptualizing a patient's experience with pain and can help to determine the appropriate treatment pathway, providers should use their clinical judgment when determining which factors to promote or discourage to optimize adaptive functioning, particularly if a patient has comorbid PTSD.

## THERAPIES FOR COMORBID CHRONIC PAIN AND POSTTRAUMATIC STRESS DISORDER

As previously described, the management of chronic pain and PTSD requires a multifactorial and interdisciplinary approach to improve patients' functional status across various domains. Among these approaches that have shown promise is mindfulness. Mindfulness originates from a Buddhist contemplative tradition and involves self-regulated attention, maintained on immediate experience, and held within an orientation of curiosity, openness, and acceptance of thoughts and emotions.[17] A 2015 meta-analysis found limited evidence for effectiveness of mindfulness-based interventions for patients with chronic pain[11]; however, a subsequent meta-analysis from 2017 showed a small decrease in pain compared with all types of controls in 30 randomized control trials (RCTs) and also found statistically significant effects for depression and quality of life.[18] The investigators cautioned, however, that additional well-designed, rigorous, and large-scale RCTs are needed to decisively provide estimates of the efficacy of mindfulness mediation for chronic pain.[18]

In addition to mindfulness, there is evidence to suggest that yoga may be beneficial in patients with chronic pain[19–21] and seems to have promising results for PTSD.[22,23] A recent study among veterans showed an overall reduction in PTSD symptoms and in symptom cluster scores of negative alterations of cognitions and mood and arousal and reactivity, in addition to reporting significant improvement in ability to participate in social activities and significant reductions in kinesiophobia (fear of movement or physical activity).[24] Of note, this particular study was limited by sample size and did have a high attrition rate of 44%. On further investigation, the investigators found that noncompleters reported significantly higher levels of anger and kinesiophobia at baseline, which may be associated with reduced ability to tolerate a group intervention, specifically one focused on slowing down and attending to internal processes such as yoga. Likewise, individuals with higher levels of kinesiophobia are likely to be more concerned about the potential harmful effects of activity.[24] This study serves as an example to illustrate the idea that although the results for many of the studies in this area skew slightly toward showing benefit while not having very large effect sizes, there are many other variables involved that may not be able to adequately capture the true impact of these interventions.

Another intervention under active investigation is pain reprocessing therapy (PRT), which aims to shift patients' beliefs about the causes and threat value of pain (accomplishes this by helping patients reconceptualize their pain as due to nondangerous brain activity rather than peripheral tissue injury, using a combination of cognitive, somatic, and exposure-based techniques).[25] A 2021 study sought to determine if PRT provides substantial and durable pain relief from chronic back pain and found that 66% of participants randomized to PRT were pain free or nearly pain free at posttreatment (reporting a pain intensity score of 0 or 1 out of 10), compared with 20% of participants randomized to placebo and 10% randomized to usual care.[25] These effects were maintained at 1-year follow-up and highlighted the fact that psychological treatment centered on changing patients' beliefs about the causes and threat value of pain may provide substantial and durable pain relief for people with chronic low back pain. It should be noted, however, that this study was not conducted in a population with comorbid PTSD.

Given the connection and feedback loop between chronic pain and mood disorders, a recent study found that implementation of a web-based self-help intervention reduced the incidence of major depressive episode onset by 52% in patients with persistent back pain, which highlights the importance of care teams being proactive in interdisciplinary approaches.[26]

Although requiring more investigation, an intervention that span across various domains is Acceptance and Commitment Therapy (ACT), which teaches patients nonjudgmental present-focused awareness of both positive and negative experiences, and encourages identification of values and the initiation of actions in line with those values.[27] A systematic review of ACT for pain demonstrated that compared with control groups, ACT patients improved psychological flexibility, pain acceptance, anxiety, depression, and functioning,[27] all of which have overlapping features with chronic pain and PTSD.

Of all the different therapeutic modalities for both chronic pain and PTSD, cognitive behavioral therapy (CBT) has the strongest evidence base.[3,5,28,29] It uses a skill-based approach that focuses on teaching patients ways to identify and change negative thoughts, feelings, and behaviors and to replace them with more adaptive strategies.[5] It has been shown through many trials to be beneficial for reducing pain, disability, and distress in chronic pain.[28] Both CBT and trauma-focused CBT (TFCBT) are effective immediately posttreatment in the treatment of PTSD; however, TFCBT may be more effective than CBT between 1 and 4 months following treatment.[29] It should be noted that both CBT and TFCBT are more effective than other therapies (supportive therapy, nondirective counseling, psychodynamic therapy, and present-centered therapy).[29]

## SUMMARY

Chronic pain is a public health problem that affects millions of people. Although pain has traditionally been associated directly with physical pathology, the cause of pain is multifactorial and must be understood through a multidimensional lens. There is a strong relationship between pain and behavioral health, specifically with PTSD. The overlap between chronic pain and PTSD must be considered when establishing treatment goals. These goals should focus on improvement in daily functioning and increasing quality of life. It is imperative for primary care providers to be acquainted with the various strategies and modalities for addressing pain in patients with mental illness.

## CLINICS CARE POINTS

- Patients suffering from chronic pain should be screened for a previous history of trauma in addition to PTSD symptoms to help elucidate treatment options.

- When counseling patients with comorbid chronic pain and PTSD, it is important to provide psychoeducation regarding the fear-avoidant (mutual maintenance) cycle to optimize perceptions about the pain, which in turn may help the patient develop insight and feel validated, each of which may contribute to increasing functional status.

- Early detection and intervention of catastrophization in a patient's thought process is critical, given its strong negative association with functioning. In addition, behavioral health referral would likely be indicated in this setting.
- Patients with comorbid chronic pain and PTSD should be provided with a CBT referral to help develop and reinforce adaptive coping strategies.

## DISCLOSURE

The authors have nothing to disclose.

## REFERENCES

1. Merskey H, Bogduk N. Classification of chronic pain. Descriptions of chronic pain syndromes and definitions of pain terms. Force on taxonomy of the International Association for the Study of Pain. Seattle (WA): IASP; 1994.
2. Turk DC. The role of psychological factors in chronic pain. Acta Anaesthesiol Scand 1999;43(9):885–8.
3. Bosco MA, Gallinati JL, Clark ME. Conceptualizing and treating comorbid chronic pain and PTSD. Pain Res Treat 2013;2013:174728.
4. Brennstuhl MJ, Tarquinio C, Montel S. Chronic pain and PTSD: evolving views on their comorbidity. Perspect Psychiatr Care 2015;51(4):295–304.
5. Kind S, Otis JD. The interaction between chronic pain and PTSD. Curr Pain Headache Rep 2019;23(12):91.
6. Elman I, Zubieta J, Borsook D. The Missing P in psychiatric training: why it is important to teach pain to psychiatrists. Arch Gen Psychiatry 2011;68(1):12–20.
7. American Psychiatric Association. Diagnostic and statistical manual of mental disorders. 5th edition. Washington (DC): Author; 2013.
8. Tesarz J, Gerhardt A, Leisner S, et al. Distinct quantitative sensory testing profiles in nonspecific chronic back pain subjects with and without psychological trauma. Pain 2015;156(4):577–86.
9. Walter S, Leissner N, Jerg-Bretzke L, et al. Pain and emotional processing in psychological trauma. Psychiatr Danub 2010;22(3):465–70.
10. Fishbain DA, Pulikal A, Lewis JE, et al. Chronic pain types differ in their reported prevalence of post -traumatic stress disorder (PTSD) and there is consistent evidence that chronic pain is associated with PTSD: an evidence-based structured systematic review. Pain Med 2017;18(4):711–35.
11. Gibson CA. Review of posttraumatic stress disorder and chronic pain: the path to integrated care. J Rehabil Res Dev 2012;49(5):753–76.
12. Bilevicius E, Sommer JL, Asmundson GJG, et al. Posttraumatic stress disorder and chronic pain are associated with opioid use disorder: results from a 2012-2013 American nationally representative survey. Drug Alcohol Depend 2018; 188:119–25.
13. Vogel M, Frank A, Choi F, et al. Chronic pain among homeless persons with mental illness. Pain Med 2017;18(12):2280–8.
14. Asmundson GJ, Bonin MF, Frombach IK, et al. Evidence of a disposition toward fearfulness and vulnerability to posttraumatic stress in dysfunctional pain patients. Behav Res Ther 2000;38(8):801–12.
15. Abdallah CG, Geha P. Chronic pain and chronic stress: two sides of the same coin? Chronic stress (thousand oaks) 2017;1. https://doi.org/10.1177/2470547017704763. 2470547017704763.

16. Jensen MP. Psychological factors the influence pain. In: Barlow DH, editor. Hypnosis for chronic pain management. New York: Oxford University Press; 2011. p. 23–35.

17. Bawa FL, Mercer SW, Atherton RJ, et al. Does mindfulness improve outcomes in patients with chronic pain? Systematic review and meta-analysis. Br J Gen Pract 2015;65(635):e387–400.

18. Hilton L, Hempel S, Ewing BA, et al. Mindfulness Meditation for Chronic Pain: Systematic Review and Meta-analysis. Ann Behav Med 2017;51(2):199–213.

19. Qaseem A, Wilt TJ, McLean RM, et al, Clinical Guidelines Committee of the American College of Physicians. Noninvasive treatments for acute, subacute, and chronic low back pain: a clinical practice guideline From the American College of Physicians. Ann Intern Med 2017;166(7):514–30.

20. Geneen LJ, Moore RA, Clarke C, et al. Physical activity and exercise for chronic pain in adults: an overview of Cochrane Reviews. Cochrane Database Syst Rev 2017;4(4):CD011279.

21. Zhu F, Zhang M, Wang D, et al. Yoga compared to non-exercise or physical therapy exercise on pain, disability, and quality of life for patients with chronic low back pain: A systematic review and meta-analysis of randomized controlled trials. PLoS One 2020;15(9):e0238544.

22. Gallegos AM, Crean HF, Pigeon WR, et al. Meditation and yoga for posttraumatic stress disorder: A meta-analytic review of randomized controlled trials. Clin Psychol Rev 2017;58:115–24.

23. Zaccari B, Callahan ML, Storzbach D, et al. Yoga for veterans with PTSD: Cognitive functioning, mental health, and salivary cortisol. Psychol Trauma 2020;12(8): 913–7.

24. Chopin SM, Sheerin CM, Meyer BL. Yoga for warriors: an intervention for veterans with comorbid chronic pain and PTSD. Psychol Trauma 2020;12(8):888–96.

25. Ashar YK, Gordon A, Schubiner H, et al. Effect of pain reprocessing therapy vs placebo and usual care for patients with chronic back pain: a randomized clinical trial. JAMA Psychiatry 2022;79(1):13–23.

26. Sander LB, Paganini S, Terhorst Y, et al. Effectiveness of a guided web-based self-help intervention to prevent depression in patients with persistent back pain: The PROD-BP randomized clinical trial. JAMA Psychiatry 2020;77(10): 1001–11.

27. Hughes LS, Clark J, Colclough JA, et al. Acceptance and Commitment Therapy (ACT) for Chronic Pain: A Systematic Review and Meta-Analyses. Clin J Pain 2017;33(6):552–68.

28. Williams ACC, Fisher E, Hearn L, et al. Psychological therapies for the management of chronic pain (excluding headache) in adults. Cochrane Database Syst Rev 2020;8(8):CD007407.

29. Bisson JI, Roberts NP, Andrew M, et al. Psychological therapies for chronic posttraumatic stress disorder (PTSD) in adults. Cochrane Database Syst Rev 2013; 2013(12):CD003388.

# Primary Care-Based Interventional Procedures for Chronic Pain

Alex McDonald, MD, CAQSM[a,b,*]

## KEYWORDS

- Primary care • Office-based • Interventional procedures for chronic pain

## KEY POINTS

- Summary of the evidence for or against different primary care-based office procedures as well as several key factors to assist clinicians in selecting patients who are most likely to benefit
- There are several tools available in the primary care setting which may be an effective part of a comprehensive pain management plan.

There are several different types of interventional therapies that can be delivered in the primary care setting. These interventions can be an effective part of a comprehensive approach to treating chronic pain and are most effective when used in conjunction with physical therapy, pharmacotherapy, and cognitive behavioral therapy, among others. It is difficult to distill the variety of interventions into a single article because these interventions vary widely based on location and pain generators; however, in this article we focus on the most commonly used interventional therapies used or available in the primary care setting.

One of the challenges of interventional therapies includes determining the best candidates as well as the best timing for these interventions. Most interventions provide temporal relief, have reduced efficacy with each subsequent intervention, and are most effective when used on conjunction with multidisciplinary treatment strategy. As such the patients who receive maximal benefit from interventional therapies often experience focal pain or specific pain generators, are engaged and committed to the treatment plan, and have appropriate expectation and well-managed mental health, which is often a

[a] Department of Family and Sports Medicine Fontana California, Southern California Permanente Medical Group; [b] Department of Family Medicine, Bernard J Tyson Kaiser Permanente School of Medicine, 9985 Sierra Avenue, Fontana, CA 92345, USA
* Department of Family Medicine, Bernard J Tyson Kaiser Permanente School of Medicine, 9985 Sierra Avenue, Fontana, CA 92345.
E-mail address: alexmmtri@gmail.com
Twitter: @alexmmtri (A.M.)

Prim Care Clin Office Pract 49 (2022) 425–437
https://doi.org/10.1016/j.pop.2022.02.002
primarycare.theclinics.com

component or subsequent issue for patients experiencing chronic pain. Patients who do not possess these characteristics, particularly those who have unrealistic expectations, poor mental health, or secondary gain, may have poor or submaximal response to interventions and in some instances may have worsening pain afterward.

Interventional targets in the primary care setting broadly include muscle, bursa, fascia, nerve, or joint. These interventions often include a variety of different medication injections, which may include steroids, local anesthetic, saline, prolotherapy, or no medication at all (dry needling), or acupuncture or transcutaneous electrical nerve stimulation (TENS). These interventions may include adjuvant modalities, such as ultrasound, to improve precision and accuracy of injection.

The choice of interventional therapy for chronic pain in the primary care setting depends highly on the clinician, location, and cause of the pain as well as a multitude of patient factors, which are discussed in this article. Furthermore, each intervention may be applied to a wide variety of pathologic conditions and anatomic locations; as such it can feel a bit overwhelming when considering what intervention should be considered. Despite widespread use of many of these therapies there is a paucity of robust high-quality studies regarding most of the interventions discussed in this article, yet the authors attempt to provide an overview of different options available to the primary care clinician as well as synthesize the evidence and expert consensus for different pain generators. Last, this article provides recommendations and specific patient factors or clinical indications that may increase the likelihood of patient benefit for each intervention, all based on the authors clinical experiences as well as synthesis of the available evidence.

Although not the focus of this article, it should be noted that pain specialists perform several more advanced interventional neuroablative or neuromodulatory procedures used to treat more widespread pain and most commonly spinal/axial pain. These procedures are beyond the scope of this article as well as the primary care setting; however, it is important to remember that additional support and treatment from interventional pain subspecialist may be available to you and your patients.

## GLUCOCORTICOIDS

Glucocorticoids have been the workhorse of interventional therapy aimed at alleviating chronic pain for decades, including but not limited to pain emanating from nerves, muscle, joints, and tendons; myofascial pain; and so on. The primary mechanism of action of glucocorticoid is a reduction in the inflammatory cascade by suppressing neutrophil cellular migration and reversal of the increased capillary permeability.

There are multiple different formulations and preparations of glucocorticoids with differences in solubility and duration of action, and in theory lower solubility will result in less systemic absorption and longer duration at the injected site; however, studies have failed to validate this theory.[1] There is no high-quality evidence to determine the superiority of one glucocorticoid over another; furthermore, there is no definitive evidence to provide guidance as to the volume and type of anesthetic to mix with glucocorticoid injection.[2] Dilution of glucocorticoid with local anesthetic often provides immediate relief and confirms placement of glucocorticoid, reduces risks of fat atrophy, and reduces possible proinflammatory effect of glucocorticoid crystal deposition (postinjection flare).[3] The most commonly used glucocorticoid preparations in the United States include triamcinolone acetonide and methylprednisolone acetate[4] generally in doses of 10 to 80 mg and 4 to 60 mg, respectively, with smaller joints and structural pathologies using the lower end of the range and larger joints using the higher doses.

Glucocorticoids typically are used for pain from joint osteoarthritis, bursitis, as well as tendinopathies, and their use is ubiquitous for osteoarthritis in the specialty and the primary care setting. However, glucocorticoids are falling out of favor for acute and chronic tendinopathies given the theoretic risk of tendon damage and lack of long-term efficacy. It is recommended that glucocorticoid injection for chronic pain due to tendinopathy be avoided[5] due to the alteration of tendon load adaptations.[6] There is evidence that long-term glucocorticoid delivery to acute tendinopathy by injection or iontophoresis dose results in short-term relief of pain and stiffness; however, without a comprehensive treatment approach to chronic tendinopathies, mechanical disruption of tendon bundle as well as symptoms persists.

The evidence of glucocorticoid injection in osteoarthritis is much better established and at this point is considered first-line treatment standard for chronic pain from osteoarthritis. The frequency and total number of corticosteroid injections that are effective and considered safe is variable, and there is no absolute number. Individual patient risk factors, as well as risks and benefits of the injection itself, need to be considered. General consensus is intra-articular glucocorticoids injections are reasonable when pain results in significant impairment of the patient's daily function or life and/or impairs their ability to effectively engage in physical therapy, weight loss, or other aspect of a comprehensive treatment plan. For osteoarthritis or bursitis, the general consensus is to wait the longest period between injections and not less than 3 months between injections. There is limited evidence that repeated glucocorticoid injections may increase the progression of cartilage thinning[7]; however, the clinical significance of these findings is not entirely care. As such glucocorticoid injections are often reserved for patients older than 50 years and/or who have moderate to serve osteoarthritic disease or significant pain. Intra-articular glucocorticoid injections specifically for pain resulting from osteoarthritis should be considered a temporizing measure. Often if the disease continues to progress these patients may consider altering their lifestyle or seek joint replacement therapy, and these treatments simply "kick the can down the road"; however, patients still benefit. Last, there is evidence that glucocorticoid injections should not be administered less than 3 months before a total joint replacement due to increased risk of surgical complication.[8] As with any treatment the risks and benefits of intra-articular glucocorticoid injections for osteoarthritic pain should be carefully considered and patient-specific factors and shared decision making should always be used.

Soft tissue and glucocorticoid injections are generally safe but can result in systemic and local adverse effects. Septic arthritis is rare and occurs in 1 in every 1000 to 3000 injections.[9] This risk can be reduced with proper skin preparation with chlorhexidine, "no touch" technique if using nonsterile gloves, cleaning vial tops with alcohol before drawing up medication, and changing needle between drawing up medicine and the injection. Infection must be distinguished from a postinjection flare. Infection typically begins 48 to 72 hours after injection, lasts days, and has crescendo and decrescendo pattern of pain, erythema, and possible systemic symptoms such as fever and malaise. In contrast, postinjection flare onset occurs less than 48 hours postinjection, begins suddenly, and only lasts a few hours. As such it is important to appropriately council patients and provide anticipatory guidance before glucocorticoid injection.

Noninfectious complications of glucocorticoid injections include tendon rupture, although this is an exceptionally rare occurrence and is associated with injection directly into the tendon, as opposed to the tendon sheath, as well as underlying tendon pathology. Nerve atrophy or necrosis can occur with injection directly into a nerve. Postinjection flare can also occur as discussed earlier. Facial flushing after glucocorticoid injection may be seen in up to 10% of individuals. It is self-limited and may be mistaken for an allergic reaction; however, it is likely not a true allergy.[2] Skin or fat atrophy as well as hypopigmentation are common with injection of superficial structures as well as individuals with darker skin pigmentation. Osteonecrosis is a rare complication of intra-articular glucocorticoid injection occurring in less than 0.1% of injections.[10] There is limited evidence that repeating glucocorticoid injections results in cartilage thinning as discussed earlier; however, this was observed on MRI, and the clinical significance of these findings is not entirely clear. Transient hyperglycemia in individuals with diabetes mellitus can occur from 1 to 2 days postinjection, and it is important to council appropriately; however, the clinical risk is often low. Last, minor bleeding or hematoma from an injection is relatively common, but almost always self-limited. Hemarthrosis or a large hematoma is a rare complication of glucocorticoid injections, and studies have demonstrated that patients on warfarin or a DOAC (Direct Oral Anti Coagulant class of drugs) are not at increased risk of major bleeding complications[11,12]; it is recommended to perform injections without interruption of anticoagulation.

Adding additional utility and accuracy to traditional anatomic-guided glucocorticoid injection in the primary care office is the use of ultrasound guidance. Traditional ultrasound machines have been large, expensive, and reserved for subspecialty proceduralists; however, over the past several years ultrasound machines are becoming increasingly smaller and more affordable for primary care office.[13] Although robust data are lacking, ultrasound may add additional therapeutic accuracy to intraarticular glucocorticoid injections, in particular the shoulder, knee, ankle, and small joints.[14,15] Furthermore, ultrasound in the primary care setting has allowed for greater and immediate access to therapeutic intervention to deeper joints with equivalent accuracy, which had traditionally required specialist referral, radiation exposure, and more expensive fluoroscopy, computed tomography, or MRI.[16,17] Examples include the hip, sacroiliac, or glenohumeral joints. Ultrasound guidance may also allow for a more precise intervention to smaller structures requiring a lower dose of glucocorticoid thereby reducing side effects. Examples include carpal tunnel or de Quervain tenosynovitis.[15] Last, ultrasound may provide benefit when patient's body habitus can make landmarks difficult to locate, and ultrasound-assisted intervention can improve the accuracy of any intervention.

Glucocorticoids have been the workhorse of chronic musculoskeletal pain and continue to be favored by many clinicians; however, in all cases the risks and benefits must be weighed. The following is a list of conditions and patient factors to consider as well as those that may increase benefit when determining if glucocorticoid is warranted in certain patients:

- Glucocorticoids are likely most appropriate for moderate to serve joint osteoarthritis
- Many clinicians reserve glucocorticoid, especially for joint injections, for those older than 50 years, or in some cases greater, due to risk of chondrocyte toxicity.
- Glucocorticoids have been shown to be beneficial in chronic bursitis that has not responded to traditional rest ice ibuprophen compression and elevation (RICE) treatments.
- Accessibility to the joint, location, and clinician training and experience as well as additional guidance, such as ultrasound, to increase accuracy may be factors when considering glucocorticoid injection.
- Glucocorticoids are falling out of favor for chronic tendinopathy, and other options should be considered first.

- Glucocorticoid injections may be considered for acute tendinopathy if immediate return of function is required; however, there are likely better first-line options.

## OTHER INJECTABLE MEDICATIONS

Hyaluronic acid and derivatives have been used to treat osteoarthritis, in particular knee joint osteoarthritis for several years; however, there is lack of robust evidence demonstrating efficacy over placebo or saline injections.[18] There are small and/or anecdotal reports of a subset of patients who benefit from intra-articular hyaluronic injections for osteoarthritis, especially if glucocorticoid no long results in clinical improvement, or younger patients with osteoarthritis; however, there are likely better options for these patients. Most experts recommend avoiding hyaluronic acid due to higher cost, increased risk of postinjection flare, and lack of robust evidence that demonstrates benefit over placebo.

Platelet-rich plasma (PRP) has garnered a significant amount of public attention due to high-profile athletes touting its benefits. PRP is created by removing a patient's whole blood and then centrifuging to separate the denser red cell from the plasma, which is then treated with a reagent further separating the buffy coat containing most of the platelets and leukocytes. There are a variety of subsequent techniques, to repeat spin (double spin) and harvest the buffy layer, which contains a higher percentage of platelet and leukocytes, or both layers to prepare for injection. The double spin technique results in a higher concentration of platelets and leukocytes often referred to as "leukocyte rich" as opposed to "leukocyte poor," which does not use the double spin technique. Emerging evidence demonstrates that leukocyte-rich PRP may be more effective when it pertains to tendinopathy treatment,[19] whereas the type of PRP for osteoarthritis is not yet clear.

PRP has been studied for various acute and chronic musculoskeletal conditions, namely, osteoarthritis and tendinopathies. The mechanism is not well understood; however, it is hypothesized to deliver concentrated growth factors triggering increased mesenchymal stem cell proliferation resulting in increased collagen and matrix synthesis. Furthermore, enhancing the expression of nuclear factor-$\kappa$B inhibitor and gene expression of interleukin-1 may reduce the inflammation of osteoarthritis by blocking downstream cytokine activation, as well as decreasing inhibition of type II collagen production.[20] The evidence is still mixed, many experts do not recommend PRP at this point, and it is often not covered by insurance. However, the number of studies demonstrating benefit of PRP and efficacy over alternatives or placebo is rapidly growing.[21] PRP studies have several limitations that make it difficult to make general recommendations. Most PRP studies are small, have limited follow-up, have multiple patient variables, and have inconsistent study design or PRP preparations or reagents, such as leuko-reduce or leukocyte rich, all of which make it difficult to draw specific conclusions.[22] Although research is still ongoing, some experts are considering PRP as a treatment option for younger patients with mild to moderate osteoarthritis, or who have failed glucocorticoid injection. Patients who may benefit most from PRP are younger patients with mild to moderate osteoarthritis. The use of PRP for chronic tendinopathies is still under investigation. However, leukocyte-rich PRP may be a good treatment option, but due to cost and lack of availability there may be better first line-treatment options.

Autologous whole blood injections (ABI) have been eclipsed by PRP injections. Original research proposed that whole blood injections promoted the growth of repair mechanisms as mentioned earlier and reduced the inflammatory cascade. However, research indicated much of these benefits were from the platelet component of ABI and as such PRP investigation followed concentrating the platelet delivered and maximized potential benefits whole reduce side effects. The advent of PPR reduced the interest, use, or research in ABI.

## Prolotherapy

Prolotherapy (or sclerotherapy) is a procedure of injecting irritants, such as dextrose, anesthetic, hypertonic saline, or a combination, into ligament or tendons to trigger an inflammatory response, which, in theory, results in strengthening of the ligaments and reduced pain. Owing to the irritant nature of prolotherapy, most patients experience a worsening of pain and function for a period of days after the procedure. This procedure is often performed in combination with trigger point injections, which may make it difficult to determine if the injection or simply the introduction of the needle results in benefit.

A systematic review compared prolotherapy, local anesthetic, and saline injections for low back pain, which resulted in no difference for short- or long-term pain relief.[23] However, there were several confounding variables in these studies, which make the results difficult to interpret. The American Pain Society recommends against prolotherapy for chronic low back pain. There have been several small studies that have examined the use of prolotherapy for chronic tendinopathy and have shown some benefit, particularly Achilles tendinopathy,[24] epicondylitis,[25] or rotator cuff syndrome.[26]

Prolotherapy may be a good option for treatment of chronic tendinopathy; however, there is no robust evidence if prolotherapy is superior to other interventions.

## Botulinum Toxin

Traditional use of Botox for chronic pain has been best studied in migraine or chronic headache. Pooled analysis of several large trials demonstrated that botulinum toxin A is modestly superior to placebo in reduction of migraine headache days but not reduction in acute headache medication use.[27–29]

Botulin toxin has also undergone some preliminary and small studies with regard to effect on chronic back pain. Botox, versus placebo, injection into paravertebral muscles resulted in superior pain relief and improved function for 50% of the participants at 3 and 8 weeks.[30] However, the benefit lasted no more than 3 to 4 months and warranted further investigation. Although there are some studies demonstrating pain relief, specifically in patients with myofascial pain syndrome, these studies are limited.[31] However, other data demonstrate no difference between botulinum toxin injection and less costly alternatives, including anesthetic, saline, or glucocorticoids[32,33]; as such Botox is not recommended for use in chronic myofascial pain.

Botulinum toxin A is beneficial in some patients who suffer from chronic migraine headache; however, due to cost, need for an experienced clinician to administer treatments, as well as limited reimbursement from insurance, botulin toxin A is recommended as a second-line medication in the treatment of chronic migraine. There is small or emerging evidence that botulinum toxin injections may benefit chronic myofascial pain or musculoskeletal back pain; however, they would not be considered first-line treatment given this limited evidence.

## Local or Trigger Point Injection

Trigger points are focal taut bands of muscle or hypersensitive nodules that are often painful to palpations and may trigger regional pain. Trigger points may be found in a variety of conditions and are commonly located in the trapezius, deep cervical, and suprascapular muscles and paraspinal or pelvic floor, although they can be located almost anywhere. Trigger points are often associated with referred pain, kinetic chain dysfunction, pain amplification, and potentially autonomic dysfunction.[34,35]

There is mixed evidence regarding the benefit of local injection of anesthetics, with or without glucocorticoids, into trigger point injections, and the procedure may provide some pain relief and is favorable given that the procedure is less dangerous or invasive than systemic medication or more invasive procedures to treat chronic pain. There are several types of medications or techniques that can be used in conjunction with trigger point injections, including choice of anesthetic, corticosteroid, saline, prolotherapy or dry needling (which are discussed elsewhere in this article), as well as the technique used to perform injection. Furthermore, it should be noted that concomitant glucocorticoid injection into musculature is falling out of favor due to lack of benefit, as well as risk of muscle necrosis.[36] There are multiple different techniques, frequency, and medication options when considering trigger point injections resulting in wide variability of data and lack of consensus or high-quality data to guide recommendations. Furthermore, there is no evidence that trigger point under ultrasound guidance improves efficacy.[37]

There is mixed or weak evidence for trigger point injection with anesthetic for both acute and chronic musculoskeletal pain. Lidocaine trigger point injections have been shown to be superior to placebo for short-term pain relief of chronic cervical pain.[38] Although limited in scope, small trials have suggested that cervical trigger point injections may reduce chronic tension-type headache frequency and abortive headache medication use.[39,40] However, a systematic review found no clear difference in short-term pain relief (1 week to 2 months) from chronic low back pain with trigger point injections using any combination of medication.[41]

Trigger point injections have also been studied in patients with chronic pelvic pain as well as myofascial pelvic pain and have demonstrated modest benefit in terms of pain reduction as well as improvement in function.[42] The most benefit was specifically for patients with relatively small and localized trigger points that reduce pain with palpation. Although pelvic trigger point injections may be referred to pelvic pain specialists, superficial or readily palpable subcutaneous trigger point injections may be performed by any clinician with knowledge of pelvic anatomy and clinical training.

There are a variety of methodical flaws and huge variability in technique and medication used within the literature examining the utility of trigger point injections. As a result, it is difficult to draw general conclusions regarding their efficacy; there is a variety of expert opinion regarding the use of trigger point injections. That being said, the risk of trigger point injections is relatively low and may be beneficial for a subset of patients, and a trial is warranted to see if there is benefit in a variety of patients. Trigger point injections are inexpensive and readily available to primary care clinicians and as such should be considered for many patients suffering from chronic myofascial or muscular pain.

Based on clinical experience here are some factors to consider and may increase the chances that trigger point injections will result in pain relief and functional improvement:

- Discrete palpable taut band of muscle or tissue that reduces pain and radiations with palpation as well as resulting in hyperactive muscle twitch response.
- Chronic or subacute tender points that have persisted for more than 6 weeks and have not responded to multiple other treatment modalities, most notably, massage, stretching, topical applications, or nonsteroidal anti-inflammatory medications.

- Able to localize trigger point and choice of needle length to be able to safely perform trigger point injection while minimizing risks to deep or surrounding anatomy, particularly neurovascular structures.
- Reduction in pain for at least 24 hours; lesser duration of pain relief indicates that repeat trigger point injections will be of limited efficacy.
- Repeated injections result in greater duration of symptom improvement with each subsequent trigger point injection being a strong indication for repeated injections. There is no evidence regarding duration between injections or total number of injections; however, injections at 2- to 4-week intervals for a total of 4 to 6 injections are generally agreed upon.
- If patient has significant improvement in pain and improvement in function for at least 3 months and then pain returns, despite continued multidisciplinary treatments (stretching, massage, heat, and range of motion), it may be reasonable to repeat a series of injections.
- If appropriate, trigger point injections should be performed with lidocaine or bupivacaine without glucocorticoids.
- There is likely increased benefit of success with trigger point injection with a total of 0.5 to 1 mL anesthetic with small aliquots injected in several different planes within each specific trigger point.
- Although studies have been limited and are unable to control for several variables and overall these studies are low quality, the data do not support widespread use of trigger point injections for chronic low back pain specifically.

## NONINJECTABLE TREATMENTS
### Dry Needling

Dry needling can take multiple forms; however, most often it involves use of a solid-bore acupuncture needle inserted into a tendon, muscle, taut band, or facial tissue at the point of maximal tenderness; the needle is then removed to the subdermis and reinserted into the structure of interest at a different plane with this process repeated over and over resulting in multiple passes or fenestration into or through the pain-generating structure. Like other interventional studies, dry needling data suffer from lack of generalizability due to the wide variety of treatment protocols, including frequency of treatment, use of ultrasound, concomitant medication injection, or clinician experience and technique. However, dry needling has been best studied in chronic tendinopathies, which have not responded to conservative treatment. In the setting of chronic tendinopathies dry needling has consistently demonstrated significant improvement in pain and return to function.[43] Dry needling can be painful, and concomitant anesthetic injection may be reasonable for those who are unable to tolerate the procedure. However, given the clinical benefit, low cost, and few adverse events, dry needling is rapidly gaining popularity as a first-line treatment of subacute or chronic tendinopathy.

Dry needling has also been investigated for use in chronic neck and myofascial pain and suffers from similar problems regarding lack of high-quality data as tendinopathy literature; however, there is emerging evidence that some patients obtain significant relief.[44,45] Given the low risk of adverse events and potential benefit, dry needling directly into taut muscle bands or local trigger points in the back or posterior neck is a reasonable option for many patients.

Dry needling is most appropriate as first-line interventional treatment of chronic tendinopathies, or myofascial trigger points that have persisted for greater then 6 to 8 weeks without response to conservative treatment options.

## Acupuncture

Acupuncture has been used as a treatment of chronic pain for thousands of years. Similar to other interventions discussed in this article, there are multiple challenges when trying to perform high-quality or randomized trial, and many sham acupuncture treatments show no benefit compared with acupuncture. However, both sham acupuncture and acupuncture treatments demonstrate significant superiority to no treatment alone in several conditions. Acupuncture treatment requires specific and additional training for primary care clinicians, which is not standard within residency; however, it may be a worthwhile service to provide patients and incorporate into one's practice.

There have been 6 high-quality randomized trials that demonstrated a small reduction in pain and improved function in patients experiencing chronic low back pain.[46] Acupuncture with sham acupuncture found some short-term reduction in pain at 6 months in patients with knee osteoarthritis.[47] It has been shown that the benefit of acupuncture in migraine and chronic tension-type headaches may be modest; however, it is a safe alternative to other treatment modalities,[48] and the UK National Institute for Health recommends acupuncture as an option when there is no response to pharmacologic treatment.

The American College of Physicians recommends acupuncture among first-line nonpharmacologic treatment of chronic pain.[49] Although there are methodical flaws, high-quality data and meta-analysis have shown that acupuncture is relatively low risk with potential benefits.[50] As such acupuncture may be a good option for patients suffering from chronic musculoskeletal pain or chronic headaches.

*Transcutaneous electrical nerve stimulation*—Although typically recommended on trial by physical therapists, there is a growing market for over-the-counter TENS device use at home or through durable medical equipment. There are limited data regarding use of TENS for chronic pain.[51] TENS applied to the skin surface delivers a low-amplitude electrical current resulting in neuromodulation for various types of chronic pain including osteoarthritis; fibromyalgia; chronic cervical, migraine, and myofascial pain; and chronic low back pain. TENS has not been rigorously studied, and often efficacy is inconclusive; however, given the availability as well as low risk of complications or side effects this may be something worth considering for your patients. The use of TENS varies dramatically given the variability of location and pain stimuli; for example, there is a small study demonstrating reduction in migraine headache days following supraorbital nerve TENS treatments[52] as opposed to application directly over the myofascial areas of tenderness. Some combine acupuncture and TENS together; however, there are little to no data regarding this approach.

## SUMMARY

Primary care physicians have multiple tools at their disposal to treat chronic pain within the office without need for referral, which can make patients save time and additional expense while also improving the satisfaction of the primary care clinician. Although there is limited evidence for several interventions for chronic pain, the long-term relationship between patient and clinician is extremely valuable when discussing treatment options and engaging in shared decision making regarding how and when interventional therapies may best be incorporated into a multidisciplinary treatment plan for chronic pain.

## CLINICS CARE POINTS

- Glucocorticoids are likely most appropriate for moderate to serve joint osteoarthritis
- Glucocorticoids have been shown to be beneficial in chronic bursitis that has not responded to traditional RICE treatments.
- Glucocorticoids should be avoided for chronic tendinopathy and other options should be considered first.
- Most experts recommend avoiding hyaluronic acid for osteoarthritis
- PRP may be beneficial for treatment of tendinopathy
- PRP may be beneficial in younger patients with mild to moderate osteoarthritis
- Prolotherapy may be a good option for treatment of chronic tendinopathy
- Botulinum toxin A is beneficial in some patients who suffer from chronic migraine headache
- Trigger point injections are a reasonable first-line intervention for discrete palpable taut band of muscle or tissue that reduces pain and radiations with palpation
- Dry needling is most appropriate as first-line interventional treatment of chronic tendinopathies, or myofascial trigger points that have persisted for greater than 6 to 8 weeks
- Acupuncture may be a good option for patients suffering from chronic musculoskeletal pain or chronic headaches

## DISCLOSURE

The authors have nothing to disclose.

## REFERENCES

1. Pyne D, Ioannou Y, Mootoo R, et al. Intra-articular steroids in knee osteoarthritis: a comparative study of triamcinolone hexacetonide and methylprednisolone acetate. Clin Rheumatol 2004;23:116.
2. Cole BJ, Schumacher HR Jr. Injectable corticosteroids in modern practice. J Am Acad Orthop Surg 2005;13:37.
3. Park KS, Peisajovich A, Michael AA, et al. Should local anesthesia be used for arthrocentesis and joint injections? Rheumatol Int 2009;29:721.
4. Centeno LM, Moore ME. Preferred intraarticular corticosteroids and associated practice: a survey of members of the American College of Rheumatology. Arthritis Care Res 1994;7:151.
5. Dean BJ, Lostis E, Oakley T, et al. The risks and benefits of glucocorticoid treatment for tendinopathy: a systematic review of the effects of local glucocorticoid on tendon. Semin Arthritis Rheum 2014;43:570.
6. Mousavizadeh R, Backman L, McCormack RG, et al. Dexamethasone decreases substance P expression in human tendon cells: an in vitro study. Rheumatology (Oxford) 2015;54:318.
7. McAlindon TE, LaValley MP, Harvey WF, et al. Effect of intra-articular triamcinolone vs saline on knee cartilage volume and pain in patients with knee osteoarthritis: a randomized clinical trial. JAMA 2017;317:1967.
8. Pereira LC, Kerr J, Jolles BM. Intra-articular steroid injection for osteoarthritis of the hip prior to total hip arthroplasty : is it safe? a systematic review. Bone Joint J 2016;98-B:1027.

9. Petersen SK, Hansen I, Andreasen RA. Low frequency of septic arthritis after arthrocentesis and intra-articular glucocorticoid injection. Scand J Rheumatol 2019; 48:393.

10. Kompel AJ, Roemer FW, Murakami AM, et al. Intra-articular Corticosteroid Injections in the Hip and Knee: Perhaps Not as Safe as We Thought? Radiology 2019; 293:656.

11. Ahmed I, Gertner E. Safety of arthrocentesis and joint injection in patients receiving anticoagulation at therapeutic levels. Am J Med 2012;125:265.

12. Yui JC, Preskill C, Greenlund LS. Arthrocentesis and joint injection in patients receiving direct oral anticoagulants. Mayo Clin Proc 2017;92:1223.

13. American College of Rheumatology Musculoskeletal Ultrasound Task Force. Ultrasound in American rheumatology practice: report of the American College of Rheumatology musculoskeletal ultrasound task force. Arthritis Care Res (Hoboken) 2010;62:1206.

14. Balint PV, Kane D, Hunter J, et al. Ultrasound guided versus conventional joint and soft tissue fluid aspiration in rheumatology practice: a pilot study. J Rheumatol 2002;29:2209.

15. Raza K, Lee CY, Pilling D, et al. Ultrasound guidance allows accurate needle placement and aspiration from small joints in patients with early inflammatory arthritis. Rheumatology (Oxford) 2003;42:976.

16. Eustace JA, Brophy DP, Gibney RP, et al. Comparison of the accuracy of steroid placement with clinical outcome in patients with shoulder symptoms. Ann Rheum Dis 1997;56:59.

17. Pourbagher MA, Ozalay M, Pourbagher A. Accuracy and outcome of sonographically guided intra-articular sodium hyaluronate injections in patients with osteoarthritis of the hip. J Ultrasound Med 2005;24:1391.

18. National Clinical Guideline Centre (UK). Osteoarthritis: care and management in adults, national institute for health and care excellence (UK), London 2014.Brown GA. AAOS clinical practice guideline: treatment of osteoarthritis of the knee: evidence-based guideline, 2nd edition. J Am Acad Orthop Surg 2013;21:577.

19. Fitzpatrick J, Bulsara M, Zheng MH. The effectiveness of platelet-rich plasma in the treatment of tendinopathy. Am J Sports Med 2017;45:226.

20. Andia I, Maffulli N. Platelet-rich plasma for managing pain and inflammation in osteoarthritis. Nat Rev Rheumatol 2013;9:721.

21. Paterson KL, Hunter DJ, Metcalf BR, et al. Efficacy of intra-articular injections of platelet-rich plasma as a symptom- and disease-modifying treatment for knee osteoarthritis - the RESTORE trial protocol. BMC Musculoskelet Disord 2018; 19:272.

22. da Costa BR, Reichenbach S, Keller N, et al. Effectiveness of non-steroidal anti-inflammatory drugs for the treatment of pain in knee and hip osteoarthritis: a network meta-analysis. Lancet 2016;387:2093.

23. Dagenais S, Yelland MJ, Del Mar C, et al. Prolotherapy injections for chronic low-back pain. Cochrane Database Syst Rev 2007;2007:CD004059.

24. Yelland MJ, Sweeting KR, Lyftogt JA, et al. Prolotherapy injections and eccentric loading exercises for painful Achilles tendinosis: a randomised trial. Br J Sports Med 2011;45:421.

25. Scarpone M, Rabago DP, Zgierska A, et al. The efficacy of prolotherapy for lateral epicondylosis: a pilot study. Clin J Sport Med 2008;18:248.

26. Bertrand H, Reeves KD, Bennett CJ, et al. Dextrose prolotherapy versus control injections in painful rotator cuff tendinopathy. Arch Phys Med Rehabil 2016;97:17.

27. Aurora SK, Dodick DW, Turkel CC, et al. OnabotulinumtoxinA for treatment of chronic migraine: results from the double-blind, randomized, placebo-controlled phase of the PREEMPT 1 trial. Cephalalgia 2010;30:793.

28. Diener HC, Dodick DW, Aurora SK, et al. OnabotulinumtoxinA for treatment of chronic migraine: results from the double-blind, randomized, placebo-controlled phase of the PREEMPT 2 trial. Cephalalgia 2010;30:804.

29. Dodick DW, Turkel CC, DeGryse RE, et al. OnabotulinumtoxinA for treatment of chronic migraine: pooled results from the double-blind, randomized, placebo-controlled phases of the PREEMPT clinical program. Headache 2010;50:921.

30. Foster L, Clapp L, Erickson M, et al. Botulinum toxin A and chronic low back pain: a randomized, double-blind study. Neurology 2001;56:1290.

31. Qerama E, Fuglsang-Frederiksen A, Kasch H, et al. A double-blind, controlled study of botulinum toxin A in chronic myofascial pain. Neurology 2006;67:241.

32. Porta M. A comparative trial of botulinum toxin type A and methylprednisolone for the treatment of myofascial pain syndrome and pain from chronic muscle spasm. Pain 2000;85:101.

33. Kamanli A, Kaya A, Ardicoglu O, et al. Comparison of lidocaine injection, botulinum toxin injection, and dry needling to trigger points in myofascial pain syndrome. Rheumatol Int 2005;25:604.

34. Giamberardino MA, Affaitati G, Fabrizio A, et al. Myofascial pain syndromes and their evaluation. Best Pract Res Clin Rheumatol 2011;25:185.

35. Lavelle ED, Lavelle W, Smith HS. Myofascial trigger points. Anesthesiol Clin 2007;25:841.

36. Labat JJ, Riant T, Lassaux A, et al. Adding corticosteroids to the pudendal nerve block for pudendal neuralgia: a randomised, double-blind, controlled trial. BJOG 2017;124:251.

37. Niraj G, Collett BJ, Bone M. Ultrasound-guided trigger point injection: first description of changes visible on ultrasound scanning in the muscle containing the trigger point. Br J Anaesth 2011;107:474.

38. Peloso P, Gross A, Haines T, et al. Medicinal and injection therapies for mechanical neck disorders. Cochrane Database Syst Rev 2007;CD000319.

39. Karadaş Ö, Inan LE, Ulaş Ü, et al. Efficacy of local lidocaine application on anxiety and depression and its curative effect on patients with chronic tension-type headache. Eur Neurol 2013;70:95.

40. Karadaş Ö, Gül HL, Inan LE. Lidocaine injection of pericranial myofascial trigger points in the treatment of frequent episodic tension-type headache. J Headache Pain 2013;14:44.

41. Staal JB, de Bie R, de Vet HC, et al. Injection therapy for subacute and chronic low-back pain. Cochrane Database Syst Rev 2008;2008:CD001824.

42. Kim DS, Jeong TY, Kim YK, et al. Usefulness of a myofascial trigger point injection for groin pain in patients with chronic prostatitis/chronic pelvic pain syndrome: a pilot study. Arch Phys Med Rehabil 2013;94:930.

43. Stoychev V, Finestone AS, Kalichman L. Dry needling as a treatment modality for tendinopathy: a narrative review. Curr Rev Musculoskelet Med 2020;13:133.

44. Esenyel M, Caglar N, Aldemir T. Treatment of myofascial pain. Am J Phys Med Rehabil 2000;79:48.

45. Alvarez DJ, Rockwell PG. Trigger points: diagnosis and management. Am Fam Physician 2002;65:653.

46. Rubinstein SM, van Middelkoop M, Kuijpers T, et al. A systematic review on the effectiveness of complementary and alternative medicine for chronic non-specific low-back pain. Eur Spine J 2010;19:1213.

47. Witt C, Brinkhaus B, Jena S, et al. Acupuncture in patients with osteoarthritis of the knee: a randomised trial. Lancet 2005;366:136.
48. Melchart D, Streng A, Hoppe A, et al. The acupuncture randomised trial (ART) for tension-type headache–details of the treatment. Acupunct Med 2005;23:157.
49. Qaseem A, Wilt TJ, McLean RM, et al. Noninvasive treatments for acute, sub-acute, and chronic low back pain: a clinical practice guideline from the american college of physicians. Ann Intern Med 2017;166:514.
50. Madsen MV, Gøtzsche PC, Hróbjartsson A. Acupuncture treatment for pain: systematic review of randomised clinical trials with acupuncture, placebo acupuncture, and no acupuncture groups. BMJ 2009;338:a3115.
51. Dailey DL, Rakel BA, Vance CG, et al. Transcutaneous electrical nerve stimulation reduces pain, fatigue and hyperalgesia while restoring central inhibition in primary fibromyalgia. Pain 2013;154:2554.
52. Schoenen J, Vandersmissen B, Jeangette S, et al. Migraine prevention with a supraorbital transcutaneous stimulator: a randomized controlled trial. Neurology 2013;80:697.

# Chronic Pain Across the Ages

Robert L. "Chuck" Rich Jr, MD[a,b,*], Robert N. Agnello, DO[b],
Garett Franklin, MD[c]

## KEYWORDS

- Chronic pain • Adult • Pediatrics • Obstetrics • Elderly

## KEY POINTS

- Chronic pain occurs across all age groups.
- Prevalence of chronic pain varies across age groups and populations.
- While there are a few painful syndromes that may occur across all age and population groups, each age and population group may have painful conditions unique to each group.
- Similarly, each age and population group may have unique physiologic considerations which may impact the expression and treatment of pain.

## INTRODUCTION

This article explores the occurrence, expression, and impact of chronic pain across the human lifespan. While pain, both acute and chronic (defined as >3 months duration) occurs more commonly as we age, chronic painful syndromes are not unique to just the older adult but can occur in the pediatric and adolescent population. Additionally, there may be physiologic factors and other considerations in a given age group and population which may impact the expression of pain and subsequently the management of chronic pain in that group although this article will not focus on pain treatment in a given group. This article begins with a discussion of chronic pain in adulthood, reviewing in sequence chronic pain in pediatrics/adolescents, the obstetric population, and then geriatrics (>65) with a review of common painful conditions unique to an age group/population and those physiologic factors which must be considered for each population.

[a] Bladen Medical Associates, Elizabethtown, 300A East McKay Street, Elizabethtown, NC 28337, USA; [b] Jerry M. Wallace School of Osteopathic Medicine, Campbell University, PO Box 4280, Buies Creek, NC 27506; [c] Cary Medical Group, 530 New Waverly Place, Suite 200, Cary, NC 27518, USA
* Corresponding author. Bladen Medical Associates, 300A East McKay Street, Elizabethtown, NC 28337.
E-mail address: robert.rich.md@gmail.com

Prim Care Clin Office Pract 49 (2022) 439–453
https://doi.org/10.1016/j.pop.2022.01.007
0095-4543/22/© 2022 Elsevier Inc. All rights reserved.
primarycare.theclinics.com

## ADULTS
### Introduction

The study of chronic pain in the adult population of 18–65 represents the gold standard of traditional chronic pain care. Pediatric, geriatric, obstetric patient, and other special pain populations do exist with their own considerations.

Chronic pain has been defined by the International Association for the Study of Pain (IASP) as pain persisting or recurring for longer than 3 months. In contrast to acute pain, which alerts individuals to potential or real tissue damage, chronic pain serves no apparent physiologic purpose and persists beyond normal healing time.[1] We will review some of the current theories of pain at the end of this section.

Chronic pain significantly impacts the everyday practice of medicine, especially in primary care with impacts on patients and the entire health care team. It is typical to evaluate a pediatric patient who is in the clinic for a wellness check who describes daily frontal one-sided headaches. Many of us have seen the adult patient that presents to the clinic as a new patient to continue chronic opioid management for a variety of pain-related issues. As primary care clinicians, we commonly see adults presenting for one complaint, whereas the underlying reason for the visit is a chronic pain complaint. Recent studies demonstrate that musculoskeletal pain conditions represent 10% to 27% of visits to primary care offices.[2–4] The most common reasons for chronic pain include low back, cervical, and headache pain.[5]

### Epidemiology

Chronic pain is ubiquitous in the world. In the United States, the incidence of chronic pain in 2019 in adults over the age of 18 was 20.5% according to recent CDC surveys.[4] Other parts of the world demonstrates similar statistics; for example, in the UK the prevalence of chronic pain ranges from 13% to 50%.[5] Further review of demographics reveals a slight difference in women (21.8%) versus men (19.1%) expression of chronic pain among those experiencing pain.[6] Regarding race, it is noted that whites report an incidence of 22.4%, African Americans 19.4%, Asians 6.4%, and Native Americans 20.2%.[4] Increasing age also demonstrates an increased incidence of chronic pain, anywhere from 9.4% in 18 to 34- year olds to 31% for those 65 and greater.[6]

### Comorbidities

It is known for decades that the occurrence of chronic pain and neuropsychiatric disease, most importantly depression, is highly comorbid.[7] On average, up to 50% of patients with some form of chronic pain display symptoms of anxiety and depression, whereas in some studies the number exceeds 75%.[8,9] Outside of mood disorders, the following comorbid conditions are also associated with chronic pain: sleep disturbance, fatigue/energy issues, and neurocognitive change. It is important to consider these comorbid conditions in crafting a skillful integrative plan of care for an individual patient. To optimize treatment response, a biopsychosocial model of care is recommended.

### The Cost

Chronic pain contributes to an estimated $560 billion each year in direct medical costs, lost productivity, and disability based on reports from 2011. These costs are estimated to exceed $635 billion per year as of 2020,[10,11] composed of direct health care costs ($261 billion to $300 billion), days of work missed ($11.6 billion to $12.7 billion), hours of work missed ($95.2 billion to $96.5 billion), and lower wages

($190.6 billion to $226.3 billion.) The cost of pain was more than that of heart disease and cancer treatments combined for the years studied.

Persons with moderate pain had annual health care expenditures $4516 higher than someone with no pain, and individuals with severe pain had costs $3210 higher than those with moderate pain. Similar differences were found for other pain conditions: $4048 higher for joint pain, $5838 for arthritis, and $9680 for functional disabilities. In addition, those with chronic pain miss a significant number of days of work compared with those that do not experience chronic pain.

## Physiology of Chronic Pain

The physiology of pain is quite complex and has been increasingly identified over the course of time but is still not completely understood. None of these theories completely accounts for chronic pain in adults, but a combination of the theories likely does help to get us close. We will review the various theories as follows.

The Specificity (or Labeled Line) Theory refers to the presence of dedicated pathways for each somatosensory modality. The fundamental tenet of the Specificity Theory is that each modality has a specific receptor and associated sensory fiber (primary afferent) that is sensitive to one specific stimulus.[12]

An Intensive (or Summation) Theory of Pain (now referred to as the Intensity Theory) has been postulated at several different times throughout history. First, conceptualized in the fourth century BC by Plato in his oeuvre Timaeus, the theory defines pain, not as a unique sensory experience but rather, as an emotion that occurs when a stimulus is stronger than usual.[12]

P. Nafe postulated a "quantitative theory of feeling," now termed the Pattern Theory of pain. This theory ignored findings of specialized nerve endings and many of the observations supporting the Specificity and/or Intensive theories of pain. The theory stated that any somaesthetic sensation occurred by a specific pattern of neural firing and that the spatial and temporal profile of firing of the peripheral nerves encoded the stimulus type and intensity. This theory added that cutaneous sensory nerve fibers, with the exception of those innervating hair cells, are the same.[12]

The most well-known theory for chronic pain is that of Melzack and Wall who proposed the Gate Control Theory of Pain in 1965. The Gate Control Theory recognized the experimental evidence that supported the Specificity and Pattern Theories and provided a model that could explain these seemingly opposed findings. In their article, Melzack and Wall carefully discussed the shortcomings of the Specificity and Pattern Theories—the two dominant theories of the era—and attempted to bridge the gap between these theories with a framework based on the aspects of each theory that had been corroborated by physiologic data. Specifically, Melzack and Wall accepted that there are nociceptors (pain fibers) and touch fibers and proposed that these fibers synapse in 2 different regions within the dorsal horn of the spinal cord: cells in the substantia gelatinosa and the "transmission" cells. The model proposed that signals produced in primary afferents from the stimulation of the skin were transmitted to 3 regions within the spinal cord: (1) the substantia gelatinosa, (2) the dorsal column, and (3) a group of cells that they called transmission cells. They proposed that the gate in the spinal cord is the substantia gelatinosa in the dorsal horn, which modulates the transmission of sensory information from the primary afferent neurons to transmission cells in the spinal cord. This gating mechanism is controlled by the activity in the large and small fibers. Large-fiber activity inhibits (or closes) the gate, whereas small-fiber activity facilitates (or opens) the gate. Activity from descending fibers that originate in supraspinal regions and project to the dorsal horn could also modulate this gate. When nociceptive information reaches a threshold that exceeds the inhibition elicited, it "opens the gate" and activates pathways that lead to the experience of pain and its related behaviors.[12]

Regardless of these theories, it would be inaccurate to package chronic pain so neatly into one of these theories mentioned above. Current research is reexamining the Labeled Line versus Pattern theory, particularly earlier in the pain response with higher order areas of the brain becoming more entwined over time as the pain becomes chronic. This discussion has highlighted the differences between the peripheral encoding of nociceptive stimuli and CNS processing and perception of pain.[12]

### Discussion

As described, the prevalence and costs of chronic pain are significant. Chronic pain at some point over a lifetime may implicate greater than 50% of people. Patients with chronic pain regularly visit primary care clinicians in a variety of settings. Health care disparity in chronic pain presents across sex, gender, and race with significant research actively ongoing in this area. Theories of chronic pain continue to evolve that will likely impact our understanding and assist in determining the way we treat adult patients with chronic pain in the future. Paying attention to this will assist in optimizing decision making. A biopsychosocial approach and the use of complementary and traditional medical care will help meet patients whereby they are in as integrative a fashion as possible.

## PEDIATRICS AND ADOLESCENTS
### Introduction

Chronic pain in the pediatric and adolescent population presents unique challenges when assessing etiology, diagnosis, management, and continuation of care as the child matures into adulthood. Pain can be characterized as persistent, as defined by > 3 months in duration, but could also be defined as recurrent or relapsing/remitting in some disease states. Etiology can be known (trauma vs nontrauma) or unknown at the time of presentation. Due to these complexities, a biopsychosocial model can be a helpful framework to view pediatric patients with chronic pain.[13]

In this model, the biological domain includes pain symptoms (intensity, characteristics, distribution) and comorbid symptoms (fatigue, function, quality of life, sleep). The psychological domain assesses emotional functioning (anxiety, depression, anger, other mood symptoms) and cognitions (coping strategies, catastrophizing, self-efficacy of pain management). Both biological and psychological domains bare resemblance to adult constructs; however, the social domain takes on another dimension in children. Parents and family dynamics must be assessed in this model given children's dependence on this environment. Family functioning, parental catastrophizing, and parental anxiety and depression play a direct role in the child's experience of pain.[14]

### Prevalence

Overall, the prevalence of chronic pain in pediatrics is much less than in adults. However, these rates increase and the predominance shifts from men to women as children mature. Certain pediatric subpopulations experience more disease burden. Evidence suggests that children suffering from chronic headaches, recurrent abdominal pain, and lower back pain more adequately reflect this population. The overall prevalence of chronic pain in these populations is between 11% and 38% based on community surveys.[15] However, some consideration should also be given to other problem-specific populations, such as postoperative patients, sickle cell disease, pediatric cancers, inflammatory and autoimmune disorders given comorbid pain can be debilitating in certain cases.

## Common Pediatric Pain Syndromes

Headaches in the pediatric population are very common. The prevalence ranges from 37% to 51% in children less than 7 years old and 57% to 82% in children up to 15 year old. Frequent headaches have been reported in 2.5% of children less than 7 years old and 15% in children up to 15 year old.[16] Interestingly, before puberty men are more affected, whereas women take on this burden moving into adulthood.[17] Headache syndromes are classified by the temporal pattern of symptoms. Acute-recurrent headaches, chronic-progressive headaches, chronic daily headaches (chronic-nonprogressive), and mixed headaches account for most patients in this population.

Acute-recurrent headaches are characterized by symptom-free intervals between headaches. Migraine with or without aura is the most common form of acute-recurrent headache with tension-type headache, cluster headache, temporomandibular joint disorder, paroxysmal hemicrania, and occipital neuralgia included as well. Pediatric migraines are polygenetic and multifactorial in nature with a primary mechanism of neural dysfunction that modulates sensitivity to excitatory and inhibitory stimuli.[18,19] The clinician's goals are to reassure the patient and family of the diagnosis and the absence of serious disease, modify triggering stimuli that affect headaches, and to provide pharmacologic and behavioral therapies to reduce disease burden and migraines episodes. Evaluation should include diet, sleep, stress, skipped meals, caffeine intake, and other medications. Treatment considerations involve analgesics such as acetaminophen, NSAIDs, triptans, and anti-emetic medications for abortive therapy. Prophylactic medications might be considered if headaches are frequently interfering with daily functioning and lifestyle.[20]

Unique to children, migraine headaches are more often experienced in bilateral frontal and temporal areas or generalized, rather than unilateral compared with adults.[21] Adolescent women experiencing migraine with aura have a slightly higher stroke risk, especially if they are taking high-dose estrogen contraceptives.[22] Progressive symptoms or comorbid neurologic abnormalities found on examination should prompt further workup into more serious etiologies.

Recurrent abdominal pain is another frequently encountered concern in the primary care office. It is defined by having at least 3 bouts of pain occurring over 3 months that are severe enough to disrupt daily activities. It accounts for 5% of primary care visits in this population.[23] Organic etiologies (gastrointestinal, genitourinary, metabolic, musculoskeletal, and neurologic) account for only about 5% to 10% of cases in children. These diagnoses should be considered when fever, vomiting, blood in stools, recurrent urinary tract infections are reported or with concerning findings on physical examination. This workup usually involves laboratory testing (CBC, CMP, ESR, CRP, pregnancy testing) or imaging (ultrasound), but more specialized tests might be used considering the potential etiology.[24]

Functional abdominal pain (nonorganic) has a 13.5% prevalence in children worldwide. Diagnosis is made clinically and standardized systems, such as the Rome IV criteria, provide some diagnostic framework. Therefore, ancillary testing should only be considered on an individual basis. Functional abdominal, not otherwise specified (NOS) accounts for 53.8%, irritable bowel syndrome 38.5%, and functional dyspepsia 7.7. %.[25] Unfortunately, 35% of children with these diagnoses meet the criteria for an adult GI disorder later in life and have other comorbid pain symptoms.[26]

Management goals are to improve the child's quality of life, reduce patient and family concerns of other serious diseases, and reduce disability from pain. Setting these expectations, rather than the elimination of pain, improve care. Cognitive-behavioral therapy and hypnotherapy reduce pain, improve quality of life, and increase remission rates.[27] Pharmacologic agents can be considered adjunctive therapy in some cases. Antacids, H2 antagonists, proton pump inhibitors might be helpful in functional dyspepsia. Guar gum, peppermint oil, and loperamide have some benefits in diarrhea predominant-IBS, whereas antispasmodics have not shown benefits. Analgesics (acetaminophen, NSAIDs) triptans, and antiemetics might be helpful in abdominal migraines for episodic pain. Prophylaxis with medications such as cyproheptadine, H1 antagonists, and propanol could be considered in abdominal migraine.[24] There is little evidence for pharmacotherapy in functional abdominal NOS.

Lower back pain is another frequent pain compliant encountered in the primary care office. Low back pain in children less than 7 years old is rare and should prompt further workup. However, the prevalence increases from 16% to 18% by 12 years old and up to 66% by 16 years of age.[28,29] History and examination are critical to making an accurate diagnosis. Imaging should be considered if the patient has any abnormal neurologic findings, nocturnal pain, radicular features, bowel incontinence, bladder retention, or pain that persists beyond 4 weeks to assess for more concerning etiologies (infectious, inflammatory, neoplastic, other anatomic etiologies). Laboratory studies (CBC, ESR, CRP, HLA-B27) might be considered if there is a concern for inflammatory conditions or neoplasm. Treatment is tailored to the etiology of disease.[30]

Lumbar muscle strain is common and related to the growth or biomechanical dysfunction of pelvis and lower extremities (tight hamstrings and quadriceps, posterior pelvic tilt). Physical therapy can be helpful to improve core strength and lower extremity flexibility. Elimination of heavy book bags has conflicting data but could be considered.

Spondylosis and spondylolisthesis are another common sets of diagnoses. They account for 6% of children with low back pain. Spondylosis is a stress fracture of the par interarticularis, whereas spondylolisthesis is the translation of the vertebral body in the setting of bilateral pars interarticularis instability. L4 (71%–95%) and L5 (5%–23%) are the most common areas affected.[31] Mechanism of injury is related to repetitive lumbar extension and pain is usually focal at the spinous process on examination. These conditions are treated with relative rest, stretching exercises, and core strengthening for about 6 weeks. 90% improve with conservative measures. MRI should only be considered after lack of progress with conservative treatments.[30] Back bracing for treatment is controversial.

Adolescent idiopathic scoliosis is another condition that occurs in about 2% to 3% of adolescents. Increasing age, severity of curvature, and injuries are linked to worsening pain. 10% to 35% of children have a comorbid condition with scoliosis such as spondylosis, spondylolisthesis, Scheuermann kyphosis, or disc herniation.[32] Treatment involves bracing and potentially surgical intervention in extreme cases. The course of treatment is guided by the severity of curvature (Cobb angle, Risser score), progression of disease, and degree of debilitation.

## Discussion

In summary, chronic pain management in children and adolescents presents unique challenges compared with adults. A biopsychosocial approach to assessment and treatment is helpful to navigate these complexities. Children experiencing headaches, chronic abdominal pain, and lower back pain warrant scrutiny as they disproportionately bear the burden of chronic pain. The clinician should focus on reducing symptom burden, improving quality of life, and addressing family concerns to effectively treat these patients.

## PREGNANT PATIENTS WITH CHRONIC PAIN
*Introduction*

The obstetric population with chronic pain is one of the least studied populations with chronic pain, with the majority of the research devoted to the pharmacologic and non-pharmacologic treatment of pain in pregnancy.[33] The presentation of the pregnant patient with chronic pain is not addressed by most obstetric references[33] yet it occurs with most pain management providers not comfortable managing the pregnant patient who is then referred back to the obstetric provider for pain care. This scenario demonstrates a clear need for team-based care with the need for increased collaboration between the pain management team and the obstetric care team.

*Prevalence*

The overall prevalence of chronic pain disorders in the pregnant population is unknown,[33] although we have clear documentation for an increased rate of opioid prescriptions written for this population over the past 2 decades.[34–37] In one study of pregnant commercial insurance beneficiaries, approximately 10% had received an opioid prescription preconception with 14.4% receiving an opioid prescription at some point in their pregnancy.[35] In that study, analysis of the data revealed marked regional variation in the opioid prescribing during pregnancy with the lowest rate noted in the Northeast and the highest in the South.[35] In another study of pregnant Medicaid recipients, the overall portion of pregnant women receiving at least one opioid prescription was 21.6% with regional variation again varying from 9.5% in the Northeast to 35.8% in the South and similarly high rates (34.0%) in the Midwest.[36] Most of the pregnant patients that were taking an opioid before pregnancy continued to do so once they became pregnant.[35]

*Common Chronic Pain Syndromes During Pregnancy*

Available data indicate that the most commonly encountered chronic pain issues in the obstetric population include various headache syndromes including migraines, back pain, abdominal pain, and joint pain including rheumatoid arthritis and sickle cell pain.[33,35–37] Similar to the overall statistics of chronic pain in pregnancy, the overall percentages for each pain syndrome remain primarily estimates with back pain the most commonly noted diagnosis followed by abdominal pain, then headaches and finally joint pain.

Back pain during pregnancy is a common occurrence, occurring primarily during the later stages of pregnancy and representing several pain generators including lumbar pain, pelvic pain, hip pain, and combinations thereof with back and pelvic pain occurring in more than 70% of pregnancies.[38] Risk factors for the occurrence of back pain in pregnancy include advancing age,[39] Caucasian and African–American race[39,40] and preexisting back pain before pregnancy including back pain during previous pregnancies.[40] Exercise, parity, and prepregnancy weight were not associated with risk.[39] The incidence of herniated discs in pregnancy is estimated to be 1 in 10,000 and is associated with typical radicular signs.[41] The occurrence of low back pain during pregnancy increases the risk of back pain in later life and subsequent pregnancies.[42]

Headaches including migraines are estimated to occur in a significant percentage although the exact prevalence in the obstetric population is unknown.[43] Pregnancy seems to be negatively associated with the risk of headaches including migraine with available evidence, suggesting that migraines occur less commonly during pregnancy.[44] Pregnant patients with headaches do seem to have an increased frequency of preterm delivery, gestational hypertension, and preeclampsia. While not focusing on the treatment of headaches in pregnancy, most resources recommend that nonpharmacologic treatments be used first before considering pharmacologic treatments with opioids last.[33]

Abdominal pain in pregnancy is a common complaint having both pregnancy and nonpregnancy-related causes. Pregnancy causes multiple anatomic, physiologic and biochemical changes which can result in abdominal pain complaints. Common pregnancy causes include round ligament pain, ectopic pregnancy, spontaneous abortion, abruption, acute fatty liver of pregnancy, uterine scar dehiscence/rupture, and chorioamnionitis with the majority of those conditions more acute than chronic.[45,46] Nonobstetric causes include gastroesophageal reflux disorder, chronic constipation, cystitis, gastritis, cholecystitis, pancreatitis, appendicitis and sickle cell crisis.[45,46] A systematic approach to abdominal pain in pregnancy must be undertaken to determine the cause including the consideration of obstetric and nonobstetric causes with testing as appropriate to establish the etiology.

### Opioids in Pregnancy

There exist a significant number of negative effects associated with the use of opioids during pregnancy, both for the pregnant mother and the infant. For the pregnant mother, studies indicate that there are higher rates of depression and anxiety as well as a higher rate of chronic medical conditions associated with opioid use during pregnancy.[47] Additionally, maternal opioid use is associated with an increased risk of preterm labor, stillbirth, and intrauterine growth retardation.[47] For the developing fetus, intrauterine opioid exposure is associated with significant risks including neonatal opioid withdrawal syndrome (NOWS) and developmental effects. Neonatal opioid withdrawal syndrome can be associated with a range of symptoms including withdrawal symptoms such as recurrent sneezing, irritability, seizures, low birth weight, feeding problems, and respiratory difficulties.[48,49] Childhood developmental issues associated with maternal opioid use include long-term effects on cognitive and motor development[50] although multiple factors including maternal and pediatric interventions may affect the expression of those outcomes.

### Discussion

The majority of the literature about pain during pregnancy has focused on the treatment of pain and the impact of those treatments including opioids on the mother and developing fetus. Chronic pain syndromes of various types do occur during pregnancy in addition to acute pain syndromes with the most common categories of pain being back pain, headaches, and abdominal pain. The various pain syndromes occurring during pregnancy may have associated long-term sequelae including the risk of ongoing chronic pain syndromes postpregnancy. The overall prevalence of all chronic pain disorders in pregnancy remains uncertain although opioid prescribing data clearly indicate a growing trend over the past decade indicative of at least an increased diagnosis of pregnancy-related pain including chronic pain. With that growing use of opioids during pregnancy there has been an increase in opioid-associated risks for both the pregnant mother and the developing fetus with the possibility of long-term complications for both mother and infant postpregnancy. With improved evaluation and management of the obstetric patent during pregnancy including lessened use of opioids, hopefully those complications can be minimized.

## THE OLDER ADULT WITH CHRONIC PAIN
### Nature of the Problem

As humans age, chronic health problems of all types multiply affecting duration and quality of life, with chronic pain of all types a significant contributor. As the elderly population (defined as adults 65+) experiences exponential growth over the succeeding decades, the occurrence of and percentages of older adults affected by chronic pain will also grow exponentially.[51] The scope of chronic pain in this population reflects a conundrum of various pain syndromes including chronic musculoskeletal pain of various types, chronic neuropathic pain of various causes, pain secondary to cancer and cancer therapies and pain associated with other chronic illnesses. Similarly, various behavioral health and social determinants of health affect the expression of chronic pain in this population and with various physiologic processes of aging also impact the expression of and ultimately the treatment of chronic pain in the elderly.

### Prevalence

Currently, over a half billion people worldwide are over the age of 65 and this number is expected to triple by 2060. Additionally, the percentage of the population over 65 is expected to make up 23.4% of the population in the US to as high as 38.8% (Japan) in other developed countries with some smaller island nations even higher.[52] Similarly, life expectancy in developed countries continues to rise with some countries expecting a rise into the 90s.[53] With advancing age, one commonly reported symptom of aging is pain with estimates ranging from 24% of this population to 72% depending on the study and data collection methods.[54–58] In one recent US study, survey data revealed that 52.9% of community-dwelling older adults reported bothersome pain within the past month. In this study group, women reported a higher occurrence of pain compared with men, whereas there was little difference in pain reported across race/ethnicity. Additionally, there was an inverse relationship of reported pain compared with educational level and a positive relationship of reported pain with comorbid conditions such as obesity, depression, or coexisting arthritis.[59] Similarly, in a study of community-dwelling adults in the US that also had a diagnosis of dementia, 63.5% of respondents experienced bothersome pain.[60]

The National Health and Aging Trends Study also revealed important information about the most common sites of pain in this age group and the co-occurrence of multiple pain sites in this study group. The most commonly reported site of pain was back pain in a third of this group with the next most common site being knee pain in one-fourth. In decreasing order of occurrence was shoulder, hip, foot, hand, and neck with the least reported sites being stomach and arm. Many patients in this study reported more than one site of pain with a fifth of study adults reporting 4 or more sites of pain. Finally, the distribution of pain sites did not vary with advancing age except for neck pain which in this study decreased with advancing age.[59]

### Epidemiology

In looking at the mechanisms, contributing factors and patient characteristics associated with the development of chronic pain in older adults, one proposed model[61] for understanding chronic pain in older adults suggested use of the Biopsychosocial (BPS) Model[62] which has already been used in other population groups for understanding chronic pain.[63,64] In using this approach, the authors of that article proposed that the interaction of biological factors, psychological factors and social factors contributed to the development of chronic pain in this population.[61] Under this proposed model, biological factors included advancing age (defined as >65), female

sex, increasing comorbid conditions, patient reports of chronic fatigue, sleep disturbance, obesity, and substance abuse disorders were reported as biologic factors
contributing to chronic pain in this population.[61] Similarly, behavioral health disorders
including depression, anxiety, stress (including stressful life events, PTSD,[65]
perceived stress[66]) are reported as reported as significant factors in the development
of chronic pain.[61] Finally, the BPS model examined the effect of socioeconomic factors associated with chronic pain in older adults noting positive relationships between
lower income/education levels,[67] social isolation and loneliness[68] and the occurrence
of chronic pain.[61]

### Geriatric Chronic Pain Pharmacology Considerations

Caring for geriatric patient with chronic pain requires a consideration of various physiologic changes which impact the choice and dosing of pharmacologic options chosen
for pain management. While this article does not outline the treatment of chronic pain
in this age group, it will briefly detail those physiologic changes affecting pain
treatment.

Commonly, as the patient with chronic pain ages, this results in reduced muscle
mass, increased body fat, and a reduction in body fluid volume.[69] This subsequently
affects the volume of distribution available to medications which can then subsequently affect the plasma levels, onset of action, and elimination of classes of medications in this age group including analgesics, antidepressants, anticonvulsants,
NSAIDs, and other pharmacologic therapies.

Advancing age is also associated with changes in hepatic and renal function which
will ultimately affect the clearance of medications. Changes in hepatic metabolism
may result in the increased bioavailability of medications requiring a reduction in
drug dosages and longer intervals between doses. Similarly, changes in renal function,
particularly glomerular filtration rate, may result in a longer half-life of medications
excreted through the kidney as well higher levels of active metabolites of medications
such as morphine.[69,70] Again these renal changes may require changes in dosages
and dosing intervals of renal excreted medications and may limit choices of adjunctive
medications such as NSAIDs which have increased risk of renal toxicity in individuals
with preexisting renal impairment. Gastrointestinal changes also occur with aging
which may result in slower gastrointestinal transit time resulting in lengthened bioavailability of continuous release medications including the continuous release forms of
opioid pain relievers.[71,72] Chronic pain in the geriatric patient is rarely the only condition being treated with the geriatric patients also receiving treatment of other comorbid
conditions. With the geriatric patient on average using 2 to 5 medications on a regular
basis,[70] there exists the possibility of drug–drug interactions which must be
accounted for in choosing medications as well as the possibility of drug–disease
interactions.[72]

### Impact of Chronic Pain in the Older Adult

Chronic pain in this age group is known to have a significant impact on physical function, cognitive function and quality of life.[61] Some of the most significant impacts of
chronic pain and its treatment in the older adult are the development of mobility issues,[73] functional disability[74] and decreased ability to perform normal activities of
daily living.[75] Both the chronic pain and the side effects of medications (dizziness, fatigue, increased fall risk) used to treat that pain contribute to the development of these
physical impairments which may affect an older person's ability to live independently.
From the perspective of cognitive impairment, the presence of chronic pain and the
use of medications such as analgesics has been positively associated with cognitive

decline in younger adults[76,77] although the effect in older adults is less certain. In limited studies, there is a suggestion that chronic pain and the use of pain medications with central nervous system effects may result in memory loss and decreased cognitive function.[78] Finally, limited studies suggest that chronic pain and presumably the treatments used to manage that chronic pain are associated with decreases in quality of life measures in this age group.[79]

## Discussion

As described above, the population of older adults is growing and for the reasons noted, the number of older adults with chronic pain will continue to grow. Many of those older adults will have more than one source of pain and may be affected by more than one type of pain. Multiple factors including underlying physical health, behavioral health, and social determinants of health will affect the expression of pain with the assumption that having more than one factor increases the likelihood of an older adult developing chronic pain and its manifestations. There are numerous physiologic factors that affect the metabolism of and associated risks with the various pharmacologic treatments used to treat pain in this age group. While this article does not address the modalities used to treat chronic pain in this age group, it does note the impact of these factors on the selection and dosages of medications typically used in pain treatment. Chronic pain in the older population and its associated treatments is clearly associated with measurable impacts including impacts on the physical and cognitive function which ultimately impact the ability of the older person to live independently. By addressing the factors which contribute to and influence the expression of chronic pain in the older person, the impact of chronic pain can hopefully be minimized, improving quality of life and the ability to maintain functional independence for a longer period of time.

## SUMMARY

This article has explored the prevalence, epidemiology, unique pain syndromes, and impact of chronic pain across the human lifespan. Each age group and that subset of the adolescent/adult female obstetric patient is affected by factors unique to that population which govern the expression of and ultimately the treatment of pain for that group. The exact prevalence of pain conditions in each group is inexact, particularly for the pediatric and obstetric groups although the available evidence indicates a growing diagnosis of chronic pain across all groups. Similarly, data suggest that the use of opioid pain relievers across all populations groups has grown substantially and with that usage, the potential complications. Clearly, more research is needed to better understand the impact of chronic pain across the human lifespan and how that pain is modulated by factors that vary by region, ethnicity, education level, and income level. By better understanding the factors which govern the experience of pain across all age and population groups, it is our hope that the occurrence of an impact by chronic pain can be lessened.

## CLINICS CARE POINTS

- The management of chronic pain across all populations should involve an integrative, team-based approach.
- Physiologic factors affecting each age group must be considered in developing a treatment plan and medication choice.

## CONFLICTS OF INTEREST

The authors have nothing to disclose.

## REFERENCES

1. Treede R-D, Rief W, Barke A, et al. Chronic pain as a symptom or a disease: the IASP classification of chronic pain for the international classification of diseases (ICD-11). Pain 2019;160:19–27.
2. Rekola KE, Keinänen-Kiukaanniemi S, Takala J. Use of primary health services in sparsely populated country districts by patients with musculoskeletal symptoms: consultations with a physician. J Epidemiol Community Health 1993;47(2):153–7.
3. Wiitavaara B, Fahlström M, Djupsjöbacka M. Prevalence, diagnostics and management of musculoskeletal disorders in primary health care in Sweden - an investigation of 2000 randomly selected patient records. J Eval Clin Pract 2017;23(2):325–32.
4. MacKay C, Canizares M, Davis AM, et al. Health care utilization for musculoskeletal disorders. Arthritis Care Res (Hoboken) 2010;62(2):161–9.
5. Mills SEE, Nicolson KP, Smith BH. Chronic pain: a review of its epidemiology and associated factors in population-based studies. Br J Anaesth 2019;123(2):e273–83.
6. Available at: https://wwwn.cdc.gov/NHISDataQueryTool/SHS_adult/index.html. Accessed September 10, 2021.
7. Desai G, T S J, G SK, et al. Disentangling comorbidity in chronic pain: A study in primary health care settings from India. PLoS One 2020;15(11):e0242865.
8. Currie SR, Wang J. More data on major depression as an antecedent risk factor for first onset of chronic back pain. Psychol Med 2005;35(9):1275–82.
9. Banks SM, Kerns RD. Explaining high rates of depression in chronic pain: A doiathesis-stress framework. Psychol Bull 1996;119:95–110.
10. Institute of Medicine. Committee on Advancing Pain Research, Care, and Education. In: Relieving pain in America: a blueprint for transforming prevention, care, education, and research. Washington, DC: National Academies Press; 2011.
11. Stearns LJ, Narang S, Albright RE Jr, et al. Assessment of health care utilization and cost of targeted drug delivery and conventional medical management vs conventional medical management alone for patients with cancer-related pain. JAMA Netw Open 2019;2(4):e191549.
12. Moayedi Massieh, Karen D. Davis; theories of pain: from specificity to gate control. J Neurophysiol 2013;109:5–12.
13. Zernikow B, Wager J, Hechler T, et al. Characteristics of highly impaired children with severe chronic pain: a 5-year retrospective study on 2249 pediatric pain patients. BMC Pediatr 2012;12:54.
14. Liossi C, Howard RF. Pediatric Chronic Pain: Biopsychosocial Assessment and Formulation. Pediatrics 2016;138(5):e20160331.
15. King S, Chambers CT, Huguet A, et al. The epidemiology of chronic pain in children and adolescents revisited: a systematic review. Pain 2011;152(12):2729–38.
16. Deubner DC. An epidemiologic study of migraine and headache in 10-20 year olds. Headache 1977;17(4):173–80.
17. Sillanpää M. Changes in the prevalence of migraine and other headaches during the first seven school years. Headache 1983;23(1):15–9.
18. Ducros A, Tournier-Lasserve E, Bousser MG. The genetics of migraine. Lancet Neurol 2002 Sep;1(5):285–93.
19. Qubty W, Patniyot I. Migraine Pathophysiology. Pediatr Neurol 2020;107:1–6.

20. Lewis DW. Headaches in children and adolescents. Am Fam Physician 2002; 65(4):625–32.
21. Dooley JM, Pearlman EM. The clinical spectrum of migraine in children. Pediatr Ann 2010;39(7):408–15.
22. Schürks M, Rist PM, Bigal ME, et al. Migraine and cardiovascular disease: systematic review and meta-analysis. BMJ 2009;339:b3914.
23. Gieteling MJ, Lisman-van Leeuwen Y, van der Wouden JC, et al. Childhood nonspecific abdominal pain in family practice: incidence, associated factors, and management. Ann Fam Med 2011;9(4):337–43.
24. Reust CE, Williams A. Recurrent abdominal pain in children. Am Fam Physician 2018 Jun 15;97(12):785–93.
25. Spee LA, Lisman-Van Leeuwen Y, Benninga MA, et al. Prevalence, characteristics, and management of childhood functional abdominal pain in general practice. Scand J Prim Health Care 2013;31(4):197–202.
26. Walker LS, Dengler-Crish CM, Rippel S, et al. Functional abdominal pain in childhood and adolescence increases risk for chronic pain in adulthood. Pain 2010; 150(3):568–72.
27. Levy RL, van Tilburg MA. Functional abdominal pain in childhood: background studies and recent research trends. Pain Res Manag 2012;17(6):413–7.
28. Calvo-Muñoz I, Gómez-Conesa A, Sánchez-Meca J. Prevalence of low back pain in children and adolescents: a meta-analysis. BMC Pediatr 2013;13:14.
29. Bernstein RM, Cozen H. Evaluation of back pain in children and adolescents. Am Fam Physician 2007;76(11):1669–76.
30. Achar S, Yamanaka J. Back pain in children and adolescents. Am Fam Physician 2020;102(1):19–28.
31. Bouras T, Korovessis P. Management of spondylolysis and low-grade spondylolisthesis in fine athletes. A comprehensive review. Eur J Orthop Surg Traumatol 2015;25(Suppl 1):S167–75.
32. Teles AR, Ocay DD, Bin Shebreen A, et al. Evidence of impaired pain modulation in adolescents with idiopathic scoliosis and chronic back pain. Spine J 2019; 19(4):677–86.
33. Ray-Griffith SL, Wendel MP, Stowe ZN, et al. Chronic pain during pregnancy: a review of the literature. Inter J Women's Health 2018;10:153–64.
34. Epstein RA, Bobo WV, Martin PR, et al. Increasing pregnancy-related use of opioid analgesics. Ann Epidemiol 2013;23(8):498–503.
35. Bateman BT, Hernandez-Diaz S, Rathmell JP, et al. Patterns of opioid utilization in a large cohort of commercial insurance beneficiaries in the United States. Anesthesiology 2014;120:1216–24.
36. Desai RJ, Hernandez-Diaz S, Bateman RT, et al. Increase in prescription opioid use during pregnancy among Medicaid-enrolled women. Obstet Gynecol 2014; 123(5):997–1002.
37. Wen X, Belviso N, Lebeau R, et al. Prescription opioid use among pregnant women enrolled in Rhode Island Medicaid. R I Med J (2013) 2013;102(6):35–40.
38. Mogren IM, Pohjanen AI. Low back pain and pelvic pain during pregnancy: prevalence and risk factors. Spine (Phila Pa 1976) 2005;30(8):983–91.
39. Wang SM, Dezinno P, Maranets I, et al. Low back pain during pregnancy: prevalence, risk factors, and outcomes. Obstet Gynecol 2004;104(1):65–70.
40. Fast A, Shapiro D, Ducommun EJ, et al. Low-back pain in pregnancy. Spine (Phila Pa 1976) 1987;12(4):368–71.
41. LaBan MM, Perrin JC, Latimer FR. Pregnancy and the herniated lumbar disc. Arch Phys Med Rehabil 1983;64(7):319–21.

42. Brynhildsen J, Hansson A, Persson A, et al. Follow-up of patients with low-back pain during pregnancy. Obstet Gynecol 1998;91(2):182–6.

43. Somerville BW. A study of migraine in pregnancy. Neurology 1972;22:824–8.

44. Granella F, Sances G, Zanferrari C, et al. Migraine without aura and reproductive life events; a clinical epidemiologic study in 1300 women. Headaches 1993; 33(7):385–9.

45. Gregory DS, Wu V, Tuladhar P. The pregnant patient: managing common acute medical problems. Am Fam Physician 2018;98(9):595–602.

46. Pinas-Carrillo A, Chandraharan E. Abdominal pain in pregnancy: a rational approach to management. Obstet Gynaecol Reprod Med 2017;27(4):112–9.

47. Whitman VE, Salemi JL, Mogos MF, et al. Maternal opioid drug use during pregnancy and its impact on perinatal morbidity, mortality, and the costs of medical care in the United States. J Pregnancy 2014;9:06723.

48. Patrick SW, Schumacher RE, Benneyworth BD, et al. Neonatal Abstinence Syndrome and associated health care expenditures United States, 2000-2009. JAMA 2012;307(18):1934–40.

49. Kocheriakota P. Neonatal Abstinence Syndrome. Pediatrics 2014;134(2): e547–61.

50. Logan BA, Brown MS, Hayes MJ. Neonatal Abstinence Syndrome: treatment and pediatric outcomes. Clin Obstet Gynecol 2013;56(1):186–92.

51. US Department of Health and Human Services. Administration on aging administration for community living. A profile of older adults 2016. Washington (DC): Department of Health and Human Services; 2016.

52. US Census Bureau. World Population by Age and Sex. 2021. Available at: https://www.census.gov/population/international/data/idb/worldpop.php.   Accessed September 15, 2021.

53. Gibson SJ, Lussier D. Prevalence and relevance of pain in older persons. Pain Med 2012;13:S23–6.

54. Anderson HI, Ejlertsson G, Lede I, et al. Chronic pain in a geographically defined general population: studies of differences in age, gender, social class, and pain localization. Clin J Pain 1993;9(3):174–82.

55. Blyth FM, March LM, Brnabic AJ, et al. Chronic pain in Australia: a prevalence study. Pain 2001;89(2–3):127–34.

56. Covinsky KE, Lindquist K, Dunlop DD, et al. Pain, functional limitations, and aging. J Am Geriatr Soc 2009;57(9):1556–61.

57. Helme RD, Gibson SJ. The epidemiology of pain in elderly people. Clin Geriatr Med 2001;17(3):417–31.

58. Jakobsson U, Klevsgard R, Westergren A, et al. Old people in pain: a comparative study. J Pain Symptom Manage 2003;26(1):625–36.

59. Patel K, Guralnik JM, Dansie EJ, et al. Prevalence and impact of pain among older adults in the United States: findings from the 2011 National Health and Aging Trends Study. Pain 2013;154(12):2649–57.

60. Hunt LJ, Covinsky KE, Yaffe K, et al. Pain in community-dwelling older adults with dementia: Results from the National Health and Aging Trends Study. J Am Geriatr Soc 2015;63(8):1503–11.

61. Miaskowski C, Blyth FM, Nicosia F, et al. A biopsychosocial model of chronic pain for older adults. Pain Med 2020;21(9):1793–805.

62. Engel GL. The need for a new medical model: a challenge for biomedicine. Science 1977;196(4286):129–36.

63. Taylor LEV, Stotts NA, Humphreys J, et al. A biopsychosocial-spiritual model of chronic pain in adults with sickle cell disease. Pain Manag Nurs 2013;14(4):287–301.

64. Baria AM, Pangarkar S, Abrams G, et al. Adaption of the biopsychosocial model of chronic noncancer pain in veterans. Pain Med 2019;20(1):14–27.

65. Pietrzak RH, Goldstein RB, Southwick SM, et al. Medical comorbidity of full and partial posttraumatic stress disorder in US adults: Results from Wave 2 of the National Epidemiologic Survey on Alcohol and Related Conditions. Psychosom Med 2011;73(8):697–707.

66. White RS, Jiang J, Hall CB, et al. Higher Perceived Stress Scale scores are associated with higher pain intensity and pain interference levels in older adults. J Am Geriatr Soc 2014;62(12):2350–6.

67. Grol-Prokopczyk H. Sociodemographic disparities in chronic pain, based on 12-year longitudinal data. Pain 2017;158(2):313–22.

68. Emerson K, Boggero I, Ostir G, et al. Pain as a risk factor for loneliness among older adults. J Aging Health 2018;30(9):948–57.

69. McCleane G. Pharmacological pain management in the elderly patient. Clin Interv Aging 2007;2(4):637–43.

70. Pergolizzi J, Boger RH, Budd K, et al. Opioids and the management of chronic severe pain in the elderly: Consensus statement of an International Expert Panel with focus on the six most often used World Health Organization Step III opioids (buprenorphine, fentanyl, hydromorphone, methadone, morphine, oxycodone). Pain Pract 2008;8(4):287–313.

71. Fine PG, Herr KA. Pharmacologic management of persistent pain in older persons. Clin Geriatr 2009;17(4):25–32.

72. Fine PG. Treatment guidelines for the pharmacological management of pain in older persons. Pain Med 2012;13:S57–66.

73. Ling SM, Fried LP, Garrett ES, et al. Knee osteoarthritis compromises early mobility function: The Women's Health and Aging Study II. J Rheumatol 2003;30(1):114–20.

74. Kovacs F, Noguera J, Abaira V, et al. The influence of psychological factors on low back pain-related disability in community dwelling older persons. Pain Med 2008;9(7):871–80.

75. Krebs EE, Paudel M, Taylor BC, et al. Association of opioids with falls, fractures and physical performance among older men with persistent musculoskeletal pain. J Gen Intern Med 2016;31(5):463–9.

76. Kendal SE, Sjogren P, Pimenta CA, et al. The cognitive effects of opioids in chronic non-cancer pain. Pain 2010;15(2):225–30.

77. Moriarty O, McGuire BE, Finn DP. The effect of pain on cognitive function: A review of clinical and preclinical research. Prog Neurobiol 2011;93(3):385–404.

78. Whitlock EI, Diaz-Ramirez LG, Glymour MM, et al. Association between persistent pain and memory decline and dementia in a longitudinal cohort of elders. JAMA Intern Med 2017;177(8):1146–53.

79. Jakobsson U, Hallberg IR. Pain and quality of life among older people with rheumatoid arthritis and/or osteoarthritis: a literature review. J Clin Nurs 2002;11(4):430–3.

# Management of Chronic Pain in Patients with Substance Use Disorders

Kellene Eagen, MD[a],*, Laurel Rabson, MD[b], Rebecca Kellum, MD[c]

### KEY WORDS

- Chronic noncancer pain • Chronic pain • Opioid use disorder
- Substance use disorder • Alcohol use disorder • Buprenorphine

### KEY POINTS

- Chronic noncancer pain (CNCP) and substance use disorders (SUDs) share neurobiologic pathways and processes.
- Patients with chronic pain should be screened for SUDs, as these conditions frequently cooccur.
- In co-occurring CNCP and SUD, if one disorder is left untreated, effective treatment of the other is less likely to be successful.
- Treatment for SUDs can occur in primary care or specialty settings.
- Patients with co-occurring SUDs and CNCP frequently face barriers and stigma that interfere with their care.

## INTRODUCTION/BACKGROUND/PREVALENCE

Providing the most effective and safest management of chronic noncancer pain (CNCP) requires an understanding of substance use disorders (SUD) owing to similarities in these neurobiological conditions. Both involve abnormal neural processes and have strong behavioral components.[1] For patients with co-occurring CNCP and SUDs, the most effective management involves treating the 2 conditions simultaneously.

As defined by the American Society of Addiction Medicine, addiction is "a treatable, chronic medical disease involving complex interactions among brain circuits, genetics, the environment, and an individual's life experiences. People with addiction use substances or engage in behaviors that become compulsive and often continue

[a] Department of Family Medicine and Community Health, University of Wisconsin Madison, 1100 Delaplaine Court, Madison, WI 53715, USA; [b] VA Interprofessional Advanced Fellowship in Addiction Treatment, William S. Middleton Memorial Veterans Hospital, 2500 Overlook Terrace, Madison, WI 53705, USA; [c] Addiction Medicine Fellowship, University of Wisconsin Madison, 1100 Delaplaine Court, Madison, WI 53715, USA
* Corresponding author.
*E-mail address:* kellene.eagen@fammed.wisc.edu

Prim Care Clin Office Pract 49 (2022) 455–468
https://doi.org/10.1016/j.pop.2022.01.008
0095-4543/22/© 2022 Elsevier Inc. All rights reserved.

despite harmful consequences."[2] Although many individuals use substances, most will not develop addiction. Therefore, it is important to understand the behaviors and symptoms around the use of drugs. The *Diagnostic and Statistical Manual of Mental Disorders* (Fifth Edition) (*DSM-V*) defines clinical criteria used to diagnose an SUD, which is reviewed later in this article.

People use substances for a variety of reasons, including to achieve euphoria or to self-manage stress, depression, anxiety, and pain. Over time, repeated use can lead to a dysregulated reward response and dependence. The primary neurotransmitter involved in the reward response is dopamine. The circumstances that determine susceptibility to addiction include genetics, psychological factors, and environmental factors.[1] Substance use can also contribute to the development of pain, both acute and chronic, further exacerbating the interactions between these conditions. Substance use carries the risk of acute injury, challenges with adherence to CNCP treatment plans, and pain associated with acute withdrawal syndromes. Unfortunately, patients with concurrent CNCP and SUD often have worse outcomes.[3]

The National Survey of Drug Use and Health (NSDUH) is a household interview survey aimed to characterize substance use and mental health conditions in the United States based on annual interviews of approximately 67,500 persons. Based on the 2019 NSDUH report for people aged 12 or older, it is estimated that 14.5 million people had a past-year alcohol use disorder (AUD); 8.3 million people had a past-year illicit drug use disorder, and 2.4 million had both AUD and an illicit drug use disorder.[4] NSDUH 2019 data noted that opioid use disorder (OUD), opioid misuse, and heroin use rates decreased as compared with the year prior; however, opioid overdose deaths increased from 2018 to 2019. Tragically, the COVID-19 pandemic has acutely worsened overdose deaths. The 12-month period ending in January 2021 reported 94,134 overdose deaths, which represented a 30% increase as compared with the year prior, and the largest number of deaths on record.[5] Although stimulants, alcohol, and benzodiazepines contribute to overdose risk, overdose deaths are primarily driven by opioid use, especially synthetic opioids. The Department of Justice and the Drug Enforcement Administration recently announced the number of fake pills containing fentanyl increased 430% since 2019 and that 4 of 10 fentanyl-containing fake pills contain a potentially lethal dose.[6] Patients should be advised about this risk of drug contamination and overdose.

Patients with SUDs encompass a diverse population marked by varying substances used. Similarly, patients with CNCP encompass a diverse population with different causes of pain. Therefore, characterizing the prevalence of co-occurring SUD with CNCP is difficult. A systematic review of literature cites an overall prevalence rate of 3% to 48% of current SUD in patients with CNCP.[7] Specific to patients receiving treatment with long-term opioid therapy (LTOT), a telephone survey of 705 patients treated in primary care and specialty care reported 26% met criteria for a current OUD versus 36% for a life-time OUD.[8] Screening for SUDs in all patients with CNCP is recommended.

Primary care clinicians will be best suited to treat pain effectively and safely with an understanding of how to screen, diagnose, and provide treatment for SUDs, whether within primary care or via referral to specialty care. Effective treatments, both pharmacologic and behavioral, exist for SUDs, which will be outlined in this article.

## PATIENT EVALUATION OVERVIEW

Because "the psychosocial and functional consequences of CNCP disorders have been well documented as having significant effects on the experience of pain, engagement with treatment, and health-related quality of life," it is important that any comprehensive assessment of CNCP includes these considerations, in addition to standard, neurobiological pain assessments, which have been covered previously in this journal issue.[9] The key psychosocial and behavioral variables (**Box 1**) that affect outcomes in CNCP are similarly impactful to outcomes in the treatment of patients who struggle with addiction.[10,11] Tools that specifically assess these variables are essential for developing pain treatment regimens that both address the vulnerabilities and build upon the protective factors in patients with comorbid CNCP and SUD.

In addition, screening for SUD should be included in the comprehensive assessment of chronic pain. Brief screening tools with high sensitivity for AUD, which are useful in the primary care setting, include the AUDIT-C (3 questions) and the Single Alcohol Screening Questionnaire (1 question). The CAGE questionnaire is no longer preferred because of limitations in identifying a use disorder and potential bias based on race, gender, and age.[12] For nonalcohol substance use, the DAST-10 is an abbreviated version of the Drug Abuse Screening Test that can be administered in approximately 5 minutes.

A positive screen in the primary care setting should be followed by a formal diagnostic assessment. The *DSM-V* outlines criteria for diagnosing an SUD (**Table 1**). The criteria can be applied to any substance. Notably, the criteria related to pharmacologic properties must be considered differently when assessing for a use disorder related to a prescribed substance (ie, prescription opioids, benzodiazepine, or stimulants). If a patient uses a prescription as intended under the guidance of a medical professional, the presence of tolerance or withdrawal does not count toward the diagnostic criteria, as these are known side effects that develop in the setting of chronic use.

When considering the diagnosis of OUD in patients prescribed opioids, it may be difficult to distinguish between dependence and a use disorder. Patients with concerning drug-related behaviors, such as requests for early refills or not taking medication as prescribed, may be driven by uncontrolled pain; therefore, these behaviors must be taken in context as they relate to the treatment of pain. These are nuanced situations that must be explored in depth to determine if OUD is present. When OUD is diagnosed in patients using prescription opioids, patients should be offered treatment.[13]

## TREATMENT OPTIONS FOR PATIENTS WITH CO-OCCURRING SUBSTANCE USE DISORDERS

The best treatment for patients with co-occurring CNCP and SUD is treatment of both conditions simultaneously. Stigma toward patients who use drugs is a frequent barrier

---

**Box 1**
**Variables affecting outcomes in chronic noncancer pain and substance use disorders**

- Mood and affect
- Coping strategies
- Beliefs and expectations
- Sleep quality
- Functional capacity
- Social support
- Psychiatric comorbidities

| Table 1 |
| --- |
| **Substance use disorder** *Diagnostic and Statistical Manual of Mental Disorders* (Fifth Edition) **criteria in the last 12 months** |

| *Impaired control* | |
| --- | --- |
| 1. Larger amounts or longer than intended | Y/N |
| 2. Persistent desire or attempts to cut down or stop | Y/N |
| 3. Excessive time using, getting, recovering | Y/N |
| 4. Craving | Y/N |
| *Social impairment* | |
| 5. Failure to fulfill a major role | Y/N |
| 6. Continued use despite social/interpersonal conflicts | Y/N |
| 7. Withdrawal from activities | Y/N |
| *Risky use* | |
| 8. Use in physically hazardous situations | Y/N |
| 9. Use despite knowing it is doing harm | Y/N |
| *Pharmacologic* | |
| 10. Tolerance[a] | Y/N |
| 11. Withdrawal[a] | Y/N |
| Severity: mild: 2–3; moderate: 4–5; severe: 6+. | Total no. Y |

*Abbreviations:* N, no; Y, yes.
[a] Pharmacologic criteria do not count toward the diagnosis of the substance in question is a prescription medication taken as prescribed.

to adequate care of their CNCP. These patients should have the same access to multimodal treatment of their pain as their peers who do not use substances. In addition, all patients with an SUD should be offered treatment for their SUD within primary care or be referred to specialty addiction care. Evidence-based treatment for SUDs varies by substance but includes behavioral interventions and/or pharmacotherapy. Primary care clinicians are encouraged to use motivational interviewing skills to engage patients around behavior change as it relates to substance use.[14] What follows are considerations for patients with specific SUDs.

## CHRONIC NONCANCER PAIN AND OPIOID USE DISORDER

Patients who meet criteria for OUD should be offered the full spectrum of nonpharmacologic and nonopioid pharmacotherapies for pain. They are at elevated risk for opioid overdose and should not be initiated on LTOT for CNCP. For patients with OUD already on prescription opioids for CNCP, best practice is to offer transition to a medication for OUD with analgesic properties, such as buprenorphine or methadone. The diagnosis of OUD should be discussed with the patient, and treatment (or referral to treatment) should be offered based on patient preference.

Many patients with OUD benefit from medications for opioid use disorder (MOUD). There are 3 Food and Drug Administration (FDA) -approved medications for moderate or severe OUD, as reviewed in **Table 2**.[15] The evidence for use of MOUD in OUD is strong with randomized clinical trials for all 3 FDA-approved medications showing reduction in illicit opioid use compared with no medication. In addition, methadone and buprenorphine treatments are associated with decreased risk for overdose

**Table 2**
**Medications for Opioid Use Disorder**

| Medication | Mechanism | Clinical Setting | Frequency | Clinical Pearls |
|---|---|---|---|---|
| Extended-release intramuscular naltrexone (380 mg) | Opioid antagonist | Office-based opioid treatment | Monthly | • Requires stopping opioids at least 7 d before initiation<br>• Blocks effects of opioids during period of action<br>• No analgesic benefit |
| Buprenorphine-naloxone sublingual (SL) and subcutaneous (SC) | Partial opioid agonist | OBOT (requires waivered prescriber)[16] | SL: Daily<br>SC: Monthly | • Dosing may be split (tid-qid) to take advantage of analgesic effect<br>• "Ceiling effect" on respiratory and CNS depression<br>• Typical buprenorphine doses range 8–24 mg daily<br>• Requires monitoring, including frequent office visits, urine drug testing, prescription drug monitoring programs review |
| Methadone | Opioid agonist | Certified opioid treatment program (OTP) | Daily | • Methadone daily for OUD is not intended or dosed to provide analgesic benefit<br>• Cannot be prescribed for OUD in primary care setting<br>• Highly structured OTP setting with observed dosing<br>• Dosing determined by OTP |

death.[16] All patients with OUD, including those on MOUD, should be offered behavioral treatments for their SUD as well; however, MOUD should not be withheld if a patient declines counseling.

Both naltrexone and buprenorphine-naloxone can be prescribed in primary care in a practice known as office-based opioid treatment (OBOT). Federal regulation restricts the prescribing of methadone for OUD to a certified opioid treatment program.[16] Prescribing naltrexone does not require specific training or licensure. Previously, the prescribing of buprenorphine-naloxone for OUD required completion of a training course and application for a treatment waiver. As of April 2021, the training course is no longer required for providers treating less than 30 patients per year, but providers must still apply for a waiver through Substance Abuse and Mental Health Services Administration (SAMHSA).[16] For those treating greater than 30 patients per year, the training course remains mandated. In the context of the United States' opioid epidemic and the fact that most patients with OUD do not access MOUD, providing buprenorphine for OUD within primary care is a patient-centered model of care with the potential to significantly improve access to treatment.[17] Additional resources to learn about buprenorphine for OUD are found in **Box 2**.

Buprenorphine is a partial opioid agonist with unique pharmacology that makes it an effective medication for OUD. Its properties include a ceiling effect on respiratory and central nervous system (CNS) depression, strong binding affinity with the mu opioid receptor, and slow dissociation from the receptor. As a result, there is a decreased risk of overdose from buprenorphine as compared with full opioid agonists. Although well known as a treatment for OUD, buprenorphine also provides effective analgesia. This makes buprenorphine an excellent choice for patients with OUD who have co-morbid CNCP. The half-life of sublingual (SL) buprenorphine is approximately 37 hours and is typically dosed once daily for OUD. Its duration of analgesia is only 6 to 8 hours; therefore, prescribing in divided doses (three times a day to four times a day) is most effective for pain control.[18]

Buprenorphine products for OUD include SL buprenorphine-naloxone, SL buprenorphine, and subcutaneous buprenorphine. In the SL form, there is minimal absorption of naloxone. Naloxone is co-formulated with buprenorphine as a deterrent against misuse (ie, intranasal or injection use), as using other than prescribed will result in precipitated withdrawal.[16]

Because of its analgesic properties, buprenorphine can be used in the absence of OUD for CNCP. As compared with full opioid agonists for CNCP, buprenorphine is considered to have a favorable safety profile, although data regarding its long-term efficacy for pain remain an area of ongoing investigation.[19] The transdermal and buccal formulations of buprenorphine are FDA approved for severe chronic pain only. They are not used for the treatment of OUD; however, the transdermal patch has been used in limited settings during the transition from full opioid agonists to SL buprenorphine as a way to minimize risk of precipitated withdrawal in the setting of co-occurring CNCP and OUD.[20] These formulations approved for pain are available in doses lower than those doses typically used for OUD. Patients with OUD and CNCP should be treated with the formulations approved for OUD. A complete review of buprenorphine for pain in the absence of OUD is not within the scope of this article.

Acute pain management for patients with OUD, including perioperative pain management, deserves special attention. These patients may require brief courses of opioids to achieve adequate analgesia. In these circumstances, it is encouraged to first optimize non–opioid pharmacotherapy, to provide structure and close follow-up, and to coordinate with all care providers.[16] Review of guidelines or consultation regarding management of MOUD for patients with acute pain is recommended.[21]

## CHRONIC NONCANCER PAIN AND ALCOHOL USE DISORDER

The relationship between CNCP and heavy alcohol use is complex and bidirectional. CNCP and AUD are common comorbidities and share many demographic and neurobiological factors.[22]

---

**Box 2**
**Buprenorphine for opioid use disorder resources**

- Providers clinical support system (PCSS)
  - https://pcssnow.org/
- American Society of Addiction Medicine (ASAM) Treatment of Opioid Use Disorder Course
  - https://elearning.asam.org/buprenorphine-waiver-course
- CA Bridge
  - https://cabridge.org/tools/resources/

Alcohol may be used by patients to manage pain, and although there are data supporting its acute analgesic effect, evidence that it alleviates CNCP is lacking. Indeed, excessive alcohol use may be involved in the chronification of pain and may promote hyperalgesia, yet pain is cited by many patients as a major driver of heavy alcohol use. CNCP is frequent among patients with AUD and is a risk factor for both development of AUD and for return to alcohol use in those in remission from AUD. AUD is also a risk factor for opioid misuse. Half of patients seeking treatment for AUD have concurrent CNCP.[23]

Chronic alcohol use may lead to painful conditions, including pancreatitis, alcohol-related neuropathy, and an increased risk for traumatic injuries. In addition, patients with AUD undergoing alcohol withdrawal often experience hyperalgesia.[24] When considering LTOT, concurrent use of alcohol should be assessed in light of the increased risk of sedation and overdose associated with simultaneous use of alcohol and opioids. Alcohol misuse is a risk factor for prescription opioid misuse included in the Opioid Risk Tool[24] and, generally, is a reason to avoid use of opioids for CNCP.

Patients with AUD should be offered treatment in a dedicated specialty addiction treatment or within primary care. Within the specialty setting, treatment options range from outpatient to inpatient with intermediary options, such as intensive outpatient and partial hospitalization. The ASAM Criteria are a useful tool developed to assist providers and patients to determine the most appropriate level of care.[25] Additional options include peer recovery coaches and peer recovery groups, such as Alcoholics Anonymous and Smart Recovery. The COVID-19 pandemic has altered the landscape of peer recovery groups, and many are now offered virtually, with groups accessible at all hours regardless of geography.

Patients with AUD may decline a higher level of care for a variety of reasons, and treatment within primary care can be just as effective as specialty care.[26] Primary care providers can provide addiction care in the form of educating about healthy drinking limits, using motivational interviewing to facilitate behavior change, and prescribing medications for AUD. If not available in primary care, referrals for behavioral health can also be made by a primary care provider. Medications as outlined in **Table 3** can be safely prescribed in primary care.[27] In addition to medications for AUD, treatment for co-occurring mental health conditions, such as anxiety, depression, and posttraumatic stress disorder, may aid in improvement of both CNCP and AUD.

Additional considerations for patients who use alcohol with CNCP include the risks of concurrent acetaminophen and nonsteroidal anti-inflammatory drug (NSAID) use. Acetaminophen used with alcohol increases the risk for hepatotoxicity, whereas NSAIDs used with alcohol increase the risk for gastrointestinal bleeding and renal injury. Patients should be advised of these risks.

## CHRONIC NONCANCER PAIN AND NICOTINE USE DISORDER

Nicotine has a mild acute analgesic effect, but chronic use is associated with increased likelihood of the development of CNCP. People who smoke have worse clinical outcomes for their CNCP compared with nonsmokers, including worse pain interference, sleep disturbances, fatigue, anger, and depression.[28] Chronic nicotine use also increases the risk for many painful conditions, including malignancies, atherosclerotic heart disease, and peripheral vascular disease.

Nicotine use should be assessed in patients with CNCP, and patients should be offered FDA-approved medications, including bupropion, varenicline, and nicotine replacement therapy. Although these medications do not directly alleviate pain, bupropion can treat co-occurring depression.

**Table 3**
**Medications for Alcohol Use Disorder**

| Medication | FDA Approved for AUD | Mechanism of Action | Analgesic Effect | Clinical Pearls |
|---|---|---|---|---|
| Naltrexone (oral and intramuscular) | Yes | Opioid antagonist (decreases pleasurable effect) | Possibly at low doses | Consider ER Naltrexone for concurrent OUD/AUD. Contraindicated with decompensated cirrhosis and acute liver injury |
| Acamprosate | Yes | Modulates neuronal excitability | None | Safe in advanced liver disease |
| Disulfiram | Yes | Blocks acetaldehyde dehydrogenase | None | Efficacy only shown with supervised dosing, significant toxicity |
| Gabapentin | No | Modulates GABA activity | FDA approved for neuropathic pain | Also used for alcohol withdrawal management |
| Topiramate | No | Modulates neuronal excitability | FDA approved for migraines | Requires slow titration, dose may be limited by side effects |
| Baclofen | No | Modulates neuronal excitability | FDA approved for spasticity | Use limited by sedation Safe in advanced liver disease |

*Detailed information on medications for AUD, including dosing, adverse effects, and contraindications, can be found In the primary reference for **Table 3**.

*Data from* Fairbanks J, Umbreit A, Kolla BP, Karpyak VM, Schneekloth TD, Loukianova LL, Sinha S. Evidence-Based Pharmacotherapies for Alcohol Use Disorder: Clinical Pearls. Mayo Clin Proc. 2020 Sep;95(9):1964 to 1977.

## CHRONIC NONCANCER PAIN AND OTHER SUBSTANCE USE DISORDERS

Stimulant, cannabis, and benzodiazepine use disorders exist among patients with CNCP and, like the previously addressed substances, should be treated simultaneously. Unfortunately, there are no FDA-approved medications to treat these disorders. Generally, the presence of an SUD makes patients poor candidates for LTOT, but the full spectrum of nonopioid pharmacologic and nonpharmacologic treatments for CNCP should be offered. Notably, of behavioral health strategies for these use disorders, contingency management has data to support its use, especially for stimulant use disorder.[29]

Effective treatment plans in the absence of pharmacotherapy should focus on include the following:

1. Stabilizing medical and psychiatric comorbidities,
2. Engaging the patient in shared decision making and motivational interviewing regarding patient goals,
3. Incorporating cognitive and behavioral strategies that increase positive reinforcement for nonsubstance using behaviors (ie, through formal Substance Use Disorder treatment as well as via employment, social, and leisure activities),
4. Addressing social determinants of health (ie, housing, transportation, health insurance), which are significant risk factors for substance use.

The issue of cannabis use is complicated by the patchwork of state laws on the legal status of medical and recreational cannabis. Information regarding the medical use of cannabis for chronic pain can be found in the article "The use of medical marijuana for chronic pain".

Among patients with CNCP on LTOT, many continue to be co-prescribed benzodiazepines despite recent recommendations against this practice.[30] Concurrent use of opioids and benzodiazepines is associated with increased risk of falls, emergency department visits, opioid overdose, and higher all-cause mortality.[31] Despite the risks of combining opioids with benzodiazepines, the FDA cautions that withholding buprenorphine treatment for OUD in patients already using benzodiazepines is not recommended, although close monitoring and efforts at risk mitigation are recommended.[32] Patients with co-occurring benzodiazepine use disorder and CNCP should be considered for referral to specialty addiction care.

## CONSIDERATIONS FOR OPIOID THERAPY IN PATIENTS WITH CHRONIC NONCANCER PAIN

Clinicians regularly face decisions about initiating or continuing opioids for CNCP for patients. Evaluating the risks for developing OUD and overdose is an important part of decision making. The Revised Opioid Risk Tool is a validated method to screen for the risk of developing OUD for patients beginning or continuing LTOT.[33] SOAPP-R (Screener and Opioid Assessment for Patients with Pain–Revised) can help predict which patients will have problematic behavior while on opioid treatment.[34] Risk mitigation strategies (**Table 4**) when using LTOT are always necessary, but especially for patients with OUD or those at elevated risk for developing OUD.

## REDUCING OR DISCONTINUING OPIOID THERAPY

Since the Centers for Disease Control and Prevention issued a Guideline for Prescribing Opioids for Chronic Pain in 2016, the United States has seen decreases in opioid prescribing, predominantly with decreases in new opioid prescriptions but also

| Table 4 | |
|---|---|
| **Strategies for mitigating risk with chronic opioid treatment** | |
| Emphasize goals of care | • Use a patient-centered approach that builds trust and reduces stigma<br>• Discuss realistic expectations about benefits of opioid therapy<br>• Individualize treatment plan to address unique patient risks |
| Provide structure | • Frequent visits and reassessments<br>• Shorter duration for refills<br>• Regular urine drug toxicology testing<br>• Use of patient agreements<br>• Partner with friends/family<br>• Check prescription drug monitoring programs |
| Focus on overdose risk | • Discuss and educate regarding risk factors with patient, including the use of other sedating substances (prescribed and unprescribed)<br>• Prescribe lowest possible morphine milligram equivalent<br>• Avoid abrupt and/or nonconsensual cessation or tapers of opioid prescription<br>• Provide naloxone education and prescription |

decreases in high morphine milligram equivalent regimens. In response to this guideline, there has been acknowledgment that the guideline is at times misapplied, and careful consideration should be taken when reducing or discontinuing opioid therapy. Although some studies show benefits of reducing or discontinuing opioids, other studies show potential serious harms, including opioid withdrawal, uncontrolled pain, overdose death, and mental health crises.[35] In 2019, the US Department of Health and Human Services Guide for Clinicians on the Appropriate Dose Reduction or Discontinuation of Long-Term Opioid Analgesics was released as a response to these concerns. This practical document guides providers through factors and strategies to consider when weighing the decision to reduce or discontinue opioids.[36]

## HARM REDUCTION

As defined by the National Harm Reduction Coalition, harm reduction is a "set of practical strategies and ideas aimed at reducing negative consequences associated with drug use." Although this philosophy originated in the addiction community, it can be applied to various conditions, including the management of CNCP.

Harm reduction strategies for patients with SUDs include the following:

- Overdose prevention (naloxone education and prescription)
- Information regarding access to sterile syringe programs
- Safe injection or use education
- Screening, prevention, and treatment of SUD-related infections, including hepatitis C, HIV, and sexually transmitted infections

Specific strategies for harm reduction for patients on LTOT include the following:

- Patient and family education regarding CNCP and treatment expectations
- Overdose prevention (naloxone education and prescription)
- Diagnosis and treatment of co-occurring SUD and mental health conditions
- Individualized tapers for those with risk > benefit, lowering/discontinuing total dosage to safer level
- Discontinuation of opioids for highest risk patients
- Avoiding combinations of sedating substances (benzodiazepines, Z drugs, alcohol)
- Lock boxes for safe storage of medications
- Safe disposal of unused prescription opioids

## STIGMA

Stigma toward people with SUDs and CNCP is widespread within health care settings and society in general.[37,38] Stigma further adds to the health disparities experienced by people of color, lower socioeconomic status, LGBTQ identities, and co-occurring mental health conditions. For patients with SUDs, stigma is known to be a major barrier to seeking or completing treatment.[39] Negative attitudes by health care professionals directly undermine a patient's self-esteem, self-efficacy, and sense of social support, all of which are key factors for improving functional outcomes in patients with both CNCP and addiction. **Table 5** contains a list of tools and concepts helpful to address stigma in health care settings.

## SUMMARY

An understanding of the risks for SUDs as well as how to diagnose and treat these disorders is essential to the safe and effective treatment of patients with CNCP. Because

**Table 5**
**Recommendations to Approach Stigma**

| Recommendation | Example |
|---|---|
| Avoid stigmatizing language | Addict, junkie, drug abuser, drug seeking, dirty/clean, noncompliance |
| Use patient-centered language | Person with SUD, harmful use, nonadherence, unexpected toxicology results |
| Correct misperceptions | • Opioid dependence does not equal OUD<br>• SUDs have genetic and neurobiological determinants and are not a matter of choice<br>• CNCP is not completely understood and may not be easily explained |

of the common neurologic pathways underlying addiction and chronic pain and common comorbid mental health and psychosocial challenges, these conditions should be treated concurrently. Depending on the setting and comfort level of the provider, primary care clinicians may have the resources to provide office-based treatment for SUDs or may consider referral to specialty treatment. An awareness of the stigma facing patients with both CNCP and SUD is important to provide compassionate, patient-centered care. Similarly, a harm reduction approach that meets a patient at their point of readiness is encouraged for individuals with SUDs.

## CLINICS CARE POINTS

- The diagnosis of a substance use disorder is marked by clinically significant impairment and should be made using *Diagnostic and Statistical Manual of Mental Disorders* criteria. Not all substance use meets criteria for a substance use disorder.

- Patients with chronic pain and opioid or alcohol use disorders should be offered medications for opioid or alcohol use disorders, respectively.

- Individualized care plans and slow opioid tapers can help avoid the serious harms associated with abrupt cessation of long-term opioid therapy.

- All patients at risk for overdose should be educated about and prescribed naloxone for overdose prevention.

- When considering long-term opioid therapy for chronic noncancer pain, patients should be assessed for risk of opioid misuse and overdose.

## DISCLOSURE

The authors have nothing to disclose.

## REFERENCES

1. Substance Abuse and Mental Health Services Administration. Managing CNCP in adults with or in recovery from substance use disorders. Treatment Improvement Protocol (TIP) Series 54. HHS Publication No. (SMA) 12-4671. Rockville, MD: Substance Abuse and Mental Health Services Administration; 2011.
2. ASAM definition of addiction. American Society of Addiction Medicine. 2019. Available at: https://www.asam.org/Quality-Science/definition-of-addiction. September 9, 2021.

3. John W, Wu L. Chronic non-cancer pain among adults with substance use disorders: prevalence, characteristics, and association with opioid overdose and health care utilization. Drug Alcohol Depend 2020;209:107902.

4. Substance Abuse and Mental Health Services Administration. Key substance use and mental health indicators in the United States: results from the 2019 National Survey on Drug Use and Health (HHS publication No. PEP20-07 01-001, NSDUH series H-55) 2020. Available at: https://www.samhsa.gov/data/. October 6,.

5. National Vital Statistics System. Provisional drug overdose death counts. Centers for Disease Control and Prevention. 2021. Available at: https://www.cdc.gov/nchs/nvss/vsrr/drug-overdose-data.htm. September 9.

6. US Drug Enforcement Administration. Department of Justice announces DEA seizures of historic amounts of deadly fentanyl-laced fake pills in public safety surge to protect us communities (Press Release No 21-944). 2021. Available at: https://www.justice.gov/opa/pr/department-justice-announces-dea-seizures-historic-amounts-deadly-fentanyl-laced-fake-pills. October 27, 2021.

7. Morasco BJ, Gritzner S, Lewis L, et al. Systematic review of prevalence, correlates, and treatment outcomes for chronic non-cancer pain in patients with co-morbid substance use disorder. Pain 2011;152(3):488–97.

8. Boscarino JA, Rukstalis MR, Hoffman SN, et al. Prevalence of prescription opioid-use disorder among CNCP patients: comparison of the DSM-5 vs. DSM-4 diagnostic criteria. J Addict Dis 2011;30(3):185–94.

9. Turk DC, Fillingim RB, Ohrbach R, et al. Assessment of psychosocial and functional impact of chronic pain. J Pain 2016;17(9 Suppl):T21–49.

10. Sliedrecht W, de Waart R, Witkiewitz K, et al. Alcohol use disorder relapse factors: a systematic review. Psychiatry Res 2019;278:97–115.

11. Ellis MS, Kasper Z, Cicero T. Assessment of chronic pain management in the treatment of opioid use disorder: gaps in care and implications for treatment outcomes. J Pain 2021;22(4):432–9.

12. Dhalla S, Kopec JA. The CAGE questionnaire for alcohol misuse: a review of reliability and validity studies. Clin Invest Med 2007;30(1):33–41.

13. Manhapra A, Arias AA, Ballantyne JC. The conundrum of opioid tapering in long-term opioid therapy for chronic pain: a commentary. Subst Abus 2018;39(2):152–61.

14. Smedslund G, Berg RC, Hammerstrom KT, et al. Motivational interviewing for substance abuse. Cochrane Database Syst Rev 2011;5:CD008063.

15. Substance Abuse and Mental Health Services Administration. Medications for opioid use disorder. Treatment Improvement Protocol (TIP) Series 63. Publication No. PEP21-02-01-002. Rockville, MD: Substance Abuse and Mental Health Services Administration; 2021.

16. Substance Abuse and Mental Health Services Administration. September 20, 2021. Available at: https://www.samhsa.gov/medication-assisted-treatment/become-buprenorphine-waivered-practitioner. October 8, 2021.

17. Wu LT, Zhu H, Swartz MS. Treatment utilization among persons with opioid use disorder in the United States. Drug Alcohol Depend 2016;169:117–27.

18. Webster L, Gudin J, Raffa RB, et al. Understanding buprenorphine for use in chronic pain: expert opinion. Pain Med 2020;21(4):714–23.

19. Aiyer R, Gulati A, Gungor S, et al. Treatment of chronic pain with various buprenorphine formulations: a systematic review of clinical studies. Anesth Analg 2018;127(2):529–38.

20. Adams KK, Machnicz M, Sobieraj DM. Initiating buprenorphine to treat opioid use disorder without prerequisite withdrawal: a systematic review. Addict Sci Clin Pract 2021;16:36.

21. Harrison TK, Kornfeld H, Aggarwal AK, et al. Perioperative considerations for the patient with opioid use disorder on buprenorphine, methadone, or naltrexone maintenance therapy. Anesthesiol Clin 2018;36(3):345–59.

22. Maleki N, Tahaney K, Thompson BL, et al. At the intersection of alcohol use disorder and CNCP. Neuropsychology 2019;33(6):795–807.

23. Robins MT, Heinricher MM, Ryabinin AE. From pleasure to pain and back again: the intricate relationship between alcohol and nociception. Alcohol 2019;54(6):625–38.

24. Webster LR, Webster RM. Predicting aberrant behaviors in opioid-treated patients: preliminary validation of the Opioid Risk Tool. Pain Med 2005;6(6):432–42.

25. What are the ASAM levels of care? American Society of Addiction Medicine. 2015. Available at: https://www.asamcontinuum.org/knowledgebase/what-are-the-asam-levels-of-care/. October 6, 2021.

26. O'Malley S, Rounsaville B, Farren C, et al. Initial and maintenance naltrexone treatment for alcohol dependence using primary care vs specialty care: a nested sequence of 3 randomized trials. Arch Inten Med 2003;163(14):1695–704.

27. Fairbanks J, Umbreit A, Kolla BP, et al. Evidence-based pharmacotherapies for alcohol use disorder: clinical pearls. Mayo Clin Proc 2020;95(9):1964–77.

28. Khan Js, Hah JM, Mackey SC. Effects of smoking on patients with CNCP: a propensity-weighted analysis on the Collaborative Health Outcomes Information Registry. Pain 2019;160(10):2374–9.

29. Prendergast M, Podus D, Finney J, et al. Contingency management for treatment of substance use disorders: a meta-analysis. Addiction 2006;101(11):1546–60.

30. Jeffrery M, Hooten W, Jena A, et al. Rates of physician coprescribing of opioids and benzodiazepines after the release of the Centers for Disease Control and Prevention Guidelines in 2016. JAMA Netw Open 2019;2(8):e19832S.

31. Yarborough BJ, Stumbo SP, Stoneburner A, et al. Correlates of benzodiazepine use and adverse outcomes among patients with CNCP on long-term opioid therapy. Pain Med 2019;20(6):1149–55.

32. U.S. Food and Drug Administration. FDA Drug Safety Communication: FDA urges caution about withholding opioid addiction medications from patients taking benzodiazepines or CNS depressants: careful medication management can reduce risks. 2017. Available at: https://www.fda.gov/drugs/drug-safety-and-availability/fda-drug-safety-communication-fda-urges-caution-about-withholding-opioid-addiction-medications. October 7, 2021.

33. Cheatle MD, Compton PA, Dhingra L, et al. Development of the revised opioid risk tool to predict opioid use disorder in patients with chronic nonmalignant pain. J Pain 2019;20(7):842–51.

34. Black RA, McCaffrey SA, Villapiano AJ, et al. Development and validation of an eight-item brief form of the SOAPP-R (SOAPP-8). Pain Med 2018;19(10):1982–7.

35. Mackey K, Anderson J, Bourne D, et al. Benefits and harms of long-term opioid dose reduction or discontinuation in patients with chronic pain: a rapid review. J Gen Intern Med 2020;35(Suppl 3):935–44.

36. U.S. Department of Health and Human Services. HHS guide for clinicians on the appropriate dosage reduction or discontinuation of long-term opioid analgesics. 2019. Available at: https://www.hhs.gov/opioids/sites/default/files/2019-10/Dosage_Reduction_Discontinuation.pdf. October 8, 2021.

37. van Boekel LC, Brouwers EP, van Weeghel J, et al. Stigma among health professionals towards patients with substance use disorders and its consequences for healthcare delivery: systematic review. Drug Alcohol Depend 2013;131(1–2): 23–35.

38. De Ruddere L, Craig KD. Understanding stigma and chronic pain: a-state-of-the-art review. Pain 2016;157(8):1607–10.

39. Kelly JF, Wakeman SE, Saitz R. Stop talking 'dirty': clinicians, language, and quality of care for the leading cause of preventable death in the United States. Am J Med 2015;128(1):8–9.

# Integrative Health Strategies to Manage Chronic Pain

Corey Fogleman, MD*, Kathryn McKenna, MD, MPH

## KEYWORDS

- Chronic pain • Integrative medicine • Complementary and alternative medicine

## KEY POINTS

- In 2016, the Centers for Disease Control and Prevention released guidelines recommending that "nonpharmacologic therapy and nonopioid pharmacologic therapy are preferred for chronic pain"
- Systematic reviews and/or practice guidelines support the use of acupuncture for the treatment of chronic back pain, chronic headache, and pain associated with osteoarthritis
- Systematic reviews reveal massage therapy improves short term pain and function and guidelines support its use for chronic back pain
- Systematic reviews reveal acupressure is feasible, effective, safe, and of low cost to treat low back pain and effective at improving pain and function in fibromyalgia

## INTRODUCTION

Chronic pain is variously defined, but in general is pain lasting greater than 3 months, or past the time of normal tissue healing.[1] Approximately 1 in 5, or 20% of the US population—representing 50 million adults—suffer from chronic pain.[2,3] Chronic pain causes limitations in daily functioning and decreased quality of life[3] in addition to increased risk of opioid dependence as well as anxiety and depression.[2] In 2016, the Centers for Disease Control and Prevention released guidelines for the management of chronic pain. The guidelines recommended that "nonpharmacologic therapy and nonopioid pharmacologic therapy are preferred for chronic pain."[4] Clinical practice guidelines from the American College of Physicians provide a strong recommendation to treat patients with chronic low back pain initially with nonpharmacologic treatment modalities.[5] Patients may pursue nonpharmacologic and adjunctive therapies independently or at the advice of their physicians. Patients often turn to complementary and alternative medicine modalities to manage pain when symptoms are not fully addressed by

Penn Medicine Lancaster General Health Family Medicine Residency Program, 555 North Duke Street PO Box 3555, Lancaster, PA 17604, USA
* Corresponding author.
*E-mail address:* Corey.fogleman@pennmedicine.upenn.edu

Prim Care Clin Office Pract 49 (2022) 469–483
https://doi.org/10.1016/j.pop.2022.01.001
0095-4543/22/© 2022 Elsevier Inc. All rights reserved.

conventional treatment options. Scientific evidence to support the use of integrative modalities to treat chronic pain continues to grow. Adjunctive therapies with evidence supporting its use in chronic pain include (but are not limited to) acupuncture, acupressure, massage, and mindfulness-based stress reduction (MBSR).

## INTEGRATIVE HEALTH STRATEGIES
### Acupuncture

Acupuncture is one of the practices used in traditional Chinese medicine in which practitioners stimulate specific points on the body—most often by inserting thin needles through the skin.[6] A long-practiced art that traces its organization to publications in the 2nd century BC, acupuncture principles are based on the concept that there is a unifying flow of energy, Qi or chi, analogous in some ways to the blood or lymphatic circulatory systems, that can be influenced by stimulating specific points on the body.[7] Within the acupuncture scope there are countless ways to use a needle, ways to combine points into protocols and ways to combine treatments with other therapies. When seeing an acupuncturist, a patient may be given the option of needle therapy, as well as cupping, spooning, moxibustion, use of heat, and massage both acupuncture points and nonacupuncture points.

There is always interest within the scientific community about whether acupuncture "works" for any one disease process or another, yet to ask such a question of all of Western medicine would be absurd; we would never say that acetaminophen's failure to control fracture-related pain represents an inadequacy of all pharmaceutical therapeutics. Acupuncture's effects include changing local blood flow, detectable change in adenosine at the local level, as well as endogenous opioid release.[8] Current evidence suggests that many factors—like expectation and belief—that are unrelated to acupuncture needling may play important roles in the beneficial effects of acupuncture on pain.[6]

Randomized controlled trials (RCTs) of acupuncture are fraught with challenges. Sham trials conducted with needles in nonacupuncture sites, or retractable needles may have some effect. A trial in which acupuncture methods are standardized sets aside the fact that most treatments are tailored to the patient's particular history and examination. On the other hand, trials in which treatments are individualized (the practitioner is "giving it their best shot") may reveal results contingent on the heterogeneity of practice, techniques, and skill. Regarding the use of acupuncture for the treatment of chronic pain conditions, it has been studied and is commonly used for the treatment of back pain, headache, and osteoarthritis and there is evidence that it has utility for fibromyalgia as well as endometriosis/dysmenorrhea.

### Acupressure

Acupressure, a type of acupuncture, originated in ancient China and is based on the activation of acupoints to correct the imbalance between Qi/chi[9]. Pressure is applied to targeted acupoints, causing endorphin release, muscle relaxation, and pain reduction at local sites and other body parts.[9,10] Acupressure is safe, low risk, and low cost; patients can be taught to apply acupressure independently with their fingers, handheld acupressure devices, or via adhesive vaccaria seeds to acupoints on the ear (auricular acupoints).[9,11] Acupressure is effective in treating both acute pain and chronic pain, at times alone and more often in combination with other interventions.[11]

### Massage

Massage therapy is defined as "the systematic manipulation of soft tissue with the hands that positively affects and promotes healing, reduces stress, enhances muscle relaxation, improves local circulation, and creates a sense of well-being."[12,13] Approximately 15% of the general United States population is estimated to use a massage practitioner during their lifetime.[14] While half of those use massage for general wellness or disease prevention, more than 40% use massage therapy for musculoskeletal related health problems—with more than 85% reporting that massage helped.[14] One study found that just over one-third of patients presenting to a massage therapist were referred by their physician; only one-half of presenting patients informed their health care provider they used massage therapy.[15]

The benefit of massage is mediated by stress reduction effects via decreased cortisol and increased activating neurotransmitters serotonin and dopamine.[16] Massage therapy also enhances local blood flow to "close the pain gate" and inhibit transmission of noxious stimuli by stimulating large nerve fibers shown to alter pain perception.[17] These physiologic changes lead to improvement in a variety of medical conditions including chronic pain. A meta-analysis of 32 randomized controlled studies of pain including musculoskeletal, headache, chronic pain, and fibromyalgia concluded that massage effectively treats pain and improves health-related quality of life as well as mood including anxiety.[12] Studies evaluating massage are often limited by performance and measurement bias given the difficulty in blinding participants to the treatment received as well as heterogeneity in massage technique, leading to low to very low quality of evidence in many systematic reviews.[18,19]

### Mindfulness-based stress reduction

Mindfulness-based stress reduction is a program initially developed by Dr. Jon Kabat-Zinn in 1979 for stress management; there is now evidence to support its use across many medical conditions.[20] The 8-week program uses mindfulness meditation to alleviate suffering associated with physical, psychosomatic, and psychiatric disorders. This mind-body modality of integrative medicine includes training in formal mindfulness meditation techniques including simple stretches and postures, body scan, gentle yoga, and sitting meditation, as well as mindful awareness training in relation to thoughts, sensations, and emotions.[21] MBSR is proposed to benefit patients suffering from chronic pain by increasing mindfulness and acceptance of pain[22].

### DISCUSSION

While it is the rare individual in today's marketplace who would forgo the opportunity to combine therapy options, given the choice and availability, complementary and integrative techniques are often reviewed as a sole option. Yet we would not advocate for knee replacement without postoperative pain control and physical therapy. Thus, in practical terms, therapies reviewed in this article may be appropriately suggested as adjunctive options that may be combined with one another, pharmaceuticals, manipulation, and other therapeutics. The following represents a review of the literature of these options for several common chronic pain syndromes.

### LOW BACK PAIN
#### Acupuncture

As of January 2020, up to 20 annual treatments of acupuncture treatments are covered as Centers for Medicare & Medicaid Services (CMS) benefit for patients with chronic low back pain.[23] This is based on a review of no fewer than 5 systematic reviews and supported by the guidance of several institutions, the conclusions of which are consistent that acupuncture helps with both pain and function, that even sham acupuncture has benefited and that this option is cost-effective.[24–31]

More recently, in a review of 33 studies (37 articles) with 8270 participants, acupuncture was more effective than no treatment in improving pain and function in the immediate term. Trials with usual care as the control showed acupuncture may not reduce pain clinically, but it can improve function immediately after sessions; it also improves physical but not mental quality of life in the short term.[32]

Further, a meta-analysis of 15 studies of ear acupuncture (auricular therapy, or AT) demonstrated it led to positive results in 80% of studies and concluded that it is a promising practice for chronic back pain in adults.[33] A separate systematic review of 8 studies involving 636 patients (some of them, the same studies) reached similar conclusions.[34] An examination of the harms of acupuncture reveals no serious harms, although such occurrences have been poorly reported.[24] Acupuncture by itself probably does not consistently improve long term function.[25]

A synthesis of 13 guidelines published in Europe, 10 of which were low risk of bias, concluded that chronic low back pain can be treated with acupuncture among other modalities, including exercise, acetaminophen or NSAIDs, manual therapy, and physical and psychological treatments.[35] The CMS guidance is consistent with those of the aforementioned American College of Physicians suggestions that low back pain is best treated using nonpharmacologic treatments including acupuncture.[5]

## Acupressure

A systematic review of 6 studies including more than 450 patients found acupressure to be feasible, effective, safe, and of low cost to treat low back pain.[36] On average, a 4 week treatment course of acupressure was found to significantly reduce low back pain and associated disability and improve sleep without significant adverse events.[36] A different systematic review found that acupressure may improve self-reported pain and functional limitations in low back pain but the heterogeneity and small number of studies resulted in low quality evidence.[37] Small RCTs have found acupressure to improve pain up to 35% and improve the fatigue often associated with low back pain[38]; when compared with formal physical therapy, acupressure leads to significantly more improvement in pain and disability, less absenteeism from work or school, and more satisfaction 6 months after treatment is completed.[39] A 4-week treatment course of auricular acupressure may improve pain immediately and effects seem to be sustained through 4 weeks of follow-up, without a significant therapeutic effect on disability level but also without serious adverse effects.[40]

## Massage

Massage is strongly recommended by the American College of Physicians as one of the nonpharmacologic treatment options for low back pain.[5] Systematic reviews have found that massage improves pain and function in adults experiencing subacute or chronic low back pain when compared with inactive controls (sham therapy, waiting list, or no therapy) less than 6 months after randomization; these results were not seen in the long term (greater than 6 months following randomization).[18,26] Massage did improve short-term pain and function[18,24,25] and pain at long-term follow-up[18] when compared with other active interventions such as manipulation, TENS, acupuncture, physical therapy, or relaxation interventions. Massage therapy is limited in that up to 25% of participants may experience increased pain intensity.[18]

## MBSR

The same guidance from the American College of Physicians strongly recommends the use of minfulness-based stress reduction (MBSR) as an initial nonpharmacologic treatment option for patients with chronic low back pain.[5] A RCT of nearly 350 (n = 342) adults with chronic low back pain found those who attended at least 6 of 8 MBSR sessions were significantly more likely to experience improvement in pain and function when compared with usual care at both 26 and 52 weeks following the intervention.[41] These significant findings were defined as pain reduction of 30% or more and greater than 30% improvement on a disability questionnaire. In this same study, patients completing MBSR training experienced a significant reduction in catastrophizing and improvements in self-efficacy, acceptance, and mindfulness up to 52 weeks following the completion of the program as compared with those receiving usual care.[22]

## CHRONIC HEADACHE
### Acupuncture

A systematic review of 13 RCTs of various complementary treatments for tension headache concluded that acupuncture should be considered as a nonpharmacological treatment.[42] Dry needling has also been shown to be beneficial in the treatment of chronic tension-type headache, improving intensity, frequency, and duration of headache.[43] However, regarding this option, there are fewer studies and no consistent systematic reviews.

Another systematic review included ear acupuncture as a treatment modality for the treatment of migraine without aura; 14 RCTs including 1155 participants were identified and the authors concluded that acupuncture was advantageous over medication in reducing the frequency of migraine and was more tolerated than medication because of less side effect reports (risk ratio (RR): = 0.29; 95% confidence interval (CI): 0.17–0.51; $P < .0001$).[44] However, the effects of AT begin to diminish 3 months after treatment is completed; yet the analysis of AT compared with pharmacologic analgesics showed no difference in the treatment of acute episodes in those with chronic pain syndrome.[44] Thus, like medication therapy, acupuncture seems to be a treatment rather than cure.

Regarding migraines, a Cochrane review suggests that acupuncture is helpful by itself or as an adjunct compared with control and sham, although sham seems to be modestly beneficial as well.[45] Adding acupuncture to other treatment, including medication, reduces the frequency of headaches; the authors concluded that acupuncture is as effective as treatment with prophylactic drugs.[45]

## FIBROMYALGIA
### Acupuncture

A meta-analysis of acupuncture for the treatment of fibromyalgia concluded that, while there is some value, it is at best modest.[46] Specifically, acupuncture improves pain and stiffness compared with no treatment, but the effect is not maintained 6 months after completing treatment. However, the evidence was somewhat stronger for AT, leading the authors to suggest the use of AT alone or with exercise and medication.[46] With regard to the question of real versus placebo effect, actual rather than sham acupuncture seems to have more lasting effects, as demonstrated in several small RCTs.[47–49]

### Acupressure

A systematic review found acupoint stimulation to be effective in treating fibromyalgia, resulting in reduced pain scores and the number of tender points when compared with conventional medications. Acupoint stimulation has no reported serious adverse events, although trials are often limited by methodological rigor.[50]

## Massage

Low to moderate-strength evidence supports the use of massage for small to moderate improvements in function and pain over the short and intermediate term with a small improvement in pain continuing into the long term.[51]

## Mindfulness-based Stress Reduction

In a study of more than 70 patients with fibromyalgia, more than half (51%) showed moderate to marked improvement in measures of global well-being, pain, sleep, fatigue, and feeling refreshed in the morning after participating in a weekly MBSR program for 10 weeks.[52] A systematic review of 3 trials were mixed in results, with some studies finding no difference and others finding small improvements in function and pain.[51] No harms were identified among patient with fibromyalgia treated with MBSR.[51]

# OSTEOARTHRITIS
## Acupuncture

Specialty guidelines were recently released recommending that acupuncture be conditionally recommended for patients with knee, hip, and/or hand osteoarthritis.[53]

The authors noted that knee osteoarthritis is the syndrome for which the greatest number of trials with the largest effect sizes has been carried out; yet there is variability in the results of RCTs and meta-analyses, likely driven, in part, by differences in the type and intensity of controls used.[53] However, positive trials and meta-analyses have also been published in a variety of other painful conditions and have indicated that acupuncture is effective for analgesia if not an improvement in function; thus, the Voting Panel's recommendation.[53]

A review of the literature shows that in a meta-analysis of acupuncture for the treatment of osteoarthritis, actual acupuncture is better than sham and much better than waiting-list controls at relieving pain; they conclude that the placebo-effect probably played a significant role.[54]

However, in a more recent and well-done RCT of 282 patients, acupuncture improved pain and function only modestly at 12 weeks, and there was no improvement versus no acupuncture at 12 months; there was no difference between actual acupuncture treatment and sham.[55] Another RCT—again published too recently to be included in the above-noted review—compared actual acupuncture and sham (nonpenetrating needles) when added to physical therapy; the authors concluded that there was no difference in improvement between groups.[56] Yet, another RCT showed AT resulted in less pain and better function compared with sham acupuncture after 8 weeks and that these effects persisted through week 26.[57]

Regarding dry needling, in an RCT of 242 participants with painful knee osteoarthritis, the addition of dry needling to exercise and body acupuncture resulted in decreased pain medication use and more patients achieving successful outcomes among those receiving dry needling.[58]

## Acupressure

An RCT of patients with knee osteoarthritis found an 8-week course of self-administered acupressure once daily on 5 days per week improved pain and function at 8 weeks.[59] These results may have been driven in part by the placebo-effect as there was no difference between actual and sham acupressure.[59]

## Massage

Evidence supporting the use of massage therapy for osteoarthritis is limited. One systematic review of 7 RCTs found low to moderate-quality evidence that massage is superior to nonactive therapies in reducing pain and improving functional outcomes such as range of motion in the affected joint, grip strength in hand arthritis, and walk time in knee arthritis[60]; thus massage may be considered as an adjunct to other modalities of treatment. Finally, an RCT of 125 adults with knee osteoarthritis undergoing a 60-minute massage once weekly for 8 weeks resulted in improved pain and function; by 4-months posttreatment, however, no effects were sustained.[61]

# DYSMENORRHEA
## Acupuncture

Acupuncture may be considered as a treatment modality for the management of primary dysmenorrhea but there is limited evidence. One RCT of 60 women showed a significant reduction in all studied variables including visual analog scale score for pain, menstrual cramps, headache, dizziness, diarrhea, faint, mood changes, tiredness, nausea, and vomiting in those receiving treatment.[62]

# SUMMARY

Acupuncture is not a panacea and in fact does not seem to work for several kinds of chronic pain. In fact, a recent review including a total of 67 RCTs regarding the treatment of neuropathic pain, very low-quality evidence demonstrated that acupuncture was ineffective.[63] There is even less data regarding the study of acupressure, massage, and MBSR.

## Future directions

Acupuncture is growing in popularity, the science suggests it has a benefit for our patients and it is increasingly covered by insurance, although access remains an issue (**Tables 1** and **2**). Further, the number of acupuncture schools in the United States has continued to grow and will so with the creation of the Accreditation Commission for Acupuncture and Oriental Medicine (ACAOM) and the Council of Colleges of Acupuncture and Oriental Medicine (CCAOM) in 1982. At present, there are approximately 50 schools either accredited by or are candidates for accreditation by ACAOM. These institutions provide education in acupuncture and Oriental medicine to thousands of students each year.[64]

| Table 1 States with greatest acupuncturist density in the United States as of January 2018 | |
| --- | --- |
| | Density |
| Hawaii | 52.82/1000 |
| Oregon | 34.88/1000 |
| Vermont | 30.79/1000 |
| California | 30.69/1000 |
| New Mexico | 330.27/1000 |

As of January 1, 2018, there were 37,886 licensed acupuncturists in the USA and a density of 11.63 acupuncturists/1000 patients. The 10 states with the largest number of acupuncturists were California, New York, Florida, Colorado, Washington, Oregon, Texas, New Jersey, Maryland, and Massachusetts.

| Table 2 | |
|---|---|
| States with fewer than 100 acupuncturists | |
| Nevada | Iowa |
| Wyoming | Arkansas |
| North Dakota | Mississippi |
| South Dakota | Alabama |
| Nebraska | Kentucky |
| Kansas | West Virginia |
| Oklahoma | Delaware |

States without acupuncture laws: Alabama, Oklahoma, and South Dakota.
*Data from* Refs.[64,66]

All of these modalities are being actively studied. For example, there are currently more than 100 clinical trials in various stages of recruitment and analysis examining the use of acupuncture to treat chronic pain.[65] Techniques being investigated include acupuncture shoes, bee venom injection, whether group therapy can be an effective care model and attempts to determine the proper duration of treatment.[65,66]

## CASES

### An example of an acupuncture treatment

A 29-year-old patient with 3 year history of frequent headaches and intolerance to prevention medicines requests complementary treatment. A referral to an acupuncturist results in a thorough history and physical examination, including questions about flavor and taste affinity. A look at the ears, tongue, and palpation of the pulses reveal that treatment to calm rising Liver fire may help.

Needle treatment may include placing needles at large intestine 11 to stomach 25 and manipulating, as well as adding Liver 2 (**Figs. 1–4**). These treatments last 15 to 20 minutes and are repeated weekly for 4 weeks, then repeated less often. In the meantime, indwelling ASP gold needles (which can stay in for up to 2 weeks) may be placed at Shen Men and Point Zero. If this treatment is not working well, alternative protocols can be attempted. For example, if it is determined that there is a tension component, palpation for trigger points in the neck may represent an opportunity for trigger point relaxation, with either needles or massage therapy.

### An example of massage therapy

A 55-year-old man with a history of right knee osteoarthritis presents to the office for follow-up. His pain was recently worsened by outside yardwork; he has been taking acetaminophen as needed a few days per week with some improvement. History and physical examination confirm there is crepitus on flexion and extension without erythema, edema, or restricted range of motion or strength. He has completed physical therapy as well as intra-articular steroid injection in the past and prefers an alternative adjunct to medical therapy. He is referred to a massage therapist. He is advised about the potential for increased pain intensity after the first session. He then returns once per week for 8 weeks. He notices progressive improvement in range of motion and time to walk short distances. Overall he experiences improved pain level, decreased limitations in his day-to-day function, and has required less analgesic medication use.

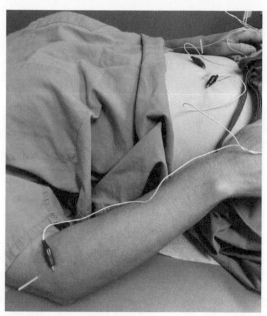

**Fig. 1.** Treatment of migraines may include Serin J type No. 3 size needles placed at Liver 11 on the arm and Stomach 25 near the navel. Treatment occurs bilaterally. Stimulation is delivered by electrical connected to transcutaneous nerve stimulation (TENS) unit and delivered for 15 minutes.

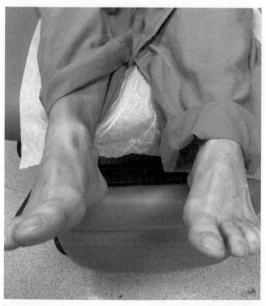

**Fig. 2.** Treatment of migraines may also include needles placed at Large Intestine 2 on the foot. Treatment occurs bilaterally.

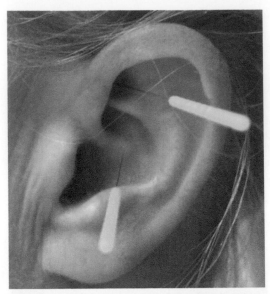

**Fig. 3.** Treatment of migraines might also include Shen Men on the triangular fossa and Point Zero on the concha. If the patient tolerates initial treatment with temporary Serin J type No. 3 size needles, usually left in for 15 minutes, ASP gold indwelling needles may be placed. The latter may stay in for a week or more, providing continuous stimulation to the acupuncture points.

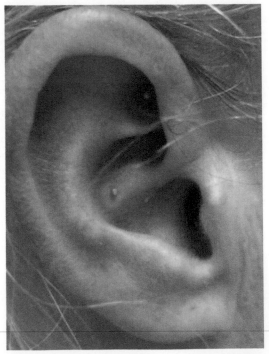

**Fig. 4.** ASP gold indwelling needles at Shen Men on the triangular fossa and Point Zero on the concha.

## An example of mindfulness-based stress reduction

A 46-year-old woman with a past medical history of anxiety, depression, and chronic low back pain presents for follow-up. She had a previous work injury and pain persisted despite the completion of physical therapy and NSAID use. She had benign imaging previously and today presents without red flags on history or physical examination that would necessitate emergent imaging or management. She has found her back pain is causing her to frequently miss work, and interrupting her ability to play comfortably with her children. This is causing her more psychological distress and interrupting her sleep. After the review of management options, you recommend enrollment into a MBSR course.

She attends 7 of the 8 sessions that occur on a weekly basis and develops improved acceptance of her pain while continuing to practice gentle yoga, stretches, and postures. Her pain and daily function improve, and although not eliminated completely, she finds her pain to be less distressing. Six months following the completion of the program, she continues to use learned techniques and finds herself more engaged at work and more active with her children at home.

## CLINICS CARE POINTS

- Acupuncture has a clear benefit for short term relief of pain in those with chronic low back pain
- Acupuncture has a clear benefit for reducing the frequency of headache in those with chronic headache
- Acupuncture has limited benefit for reducing pain in those with fibromyalgia
- Acupuncture has some value in reducing pain but not improving function in those with osteoarthritis
- Massage improves short term pain and function in patients with chronic low back pain
- Massage has some limited value for patients with fibromyalgia
- Acupressure has a benefit for short term pain relief in those with chronic low back pain
- Acupressure has no side effects and has some benefit for reducing pain in patients with fibromyalgia

## DISCLOSURE

The authors have nothing to disclose.

## REFERENCES

1. International Association for the Study of Pain. Classification of chronic pain. Descriptions of chronic pain syndromes and definitions of pain terms. Prepared by the International Association for the Study of Pain, Subcommittee on Taxonomy. Pain Suppl 1986;3:S1–226.
2. Dahlhamer J, Lucas J, Zelaya C, et al. Prevalence of Chronic Pain and High-Impact Chronic Pain Among Adults — United States, 2016. MMWR Morb Mortal Wkly Rep 2018;67:1001–6.
3. Yong RJ, Mullins P, Bhattacharyya N. Prevalence of chronic pain among adults in the United States. PAIN 2021. https://doi.org/10.1097/j.pain.0000000000002291.

4. Dowell D, Haegerich TM, Chou R. CDC Guideline for Prescribing Opioids for Chronic Pain — United States, 2016. MMWR Recomm Rep 2016;65(No. RR-1):1–49.

5. Qaseem A, Wilt TJ, McLean RM, et al. Noninvasive Treatments for Acute, Subacute and Chronic Low Back Pain: A Clinical Guideline from the American College of Physicians. Ann Intern Med 2017;166(7):514–30.

6. Available at: https://www.nccih.nih.gov/health/acupuncture-in-depth. Accessed October 29 2021.

7. Helms Joseph M. An Overview of Medical Acupuncture. In: Jonas WB, Levin JS, editors. Alternative therapies Modified from Essentials of complementary and alternative medicine, 4. Baltimore, Md: Williams & Wilkins; 1998. Available at: http://www.hmieducation.com/members/PDF/Helms%20Overview%20of%20Med%20Acu.pdf. NO. 3 35.

8. White A, Cummings TM, Filshie J. An introduction to Western medical acupuncture. Edinburgh: Churchill Livingstone/Elsevier; 2008.

9. Mehta P, Dhapte V, Kadam S, et al. Contemporary acupressure therapy: Adroit cure for painless recovery of therapeutic ailments. J Tradit Complement Med 2016;7(2):251–63.

10. Movahedi M, Ghafari S, Nazari F, et al. The Effects of Acupressure on Pain Severity in Female Nurses with Chronic Low Back Pain. Iran J Nurs Midwifery Res 2017;22(5):339–42.

11. Liu M, Tong Y, Chai L. Effects of Auricular Point Acupressure on Pain Relief: A Systematic Review. Pain Manag Nurs 2020;S1524-9042(20):30168–75.

12. Crawford C, Boyd C, Paat CF, et al. Evidence for Massage Therapy (EMT) Working Group. The impact of massage therapy on function in pain populations - a systematic review and meta-analysis of randomized controlled trials: part I, patients experiencing pain in the general population. Pain Med 2016;17(7):1353–75.

13. Sherman K, Dixon M, Thompson D, et al. Development of a taxonomy to describe massage treatment for musculoskeletal pain. BMC Complement Altern Med 2006;6(24):6–24.

14. Sundberg T, Cramer H, Sibbritt D, et al. Prevalence, patterns, and predictors of massage practitioner utilization: Results of a US nationally representative survey. Musculoskelet Sci Pract 2017;32:31–7.

15. Mastnardo D, Rose JC, Dolata J, et al. Medical Provider Recommendations to Massage Therapy: a Card Study. Int J Ther Massage Bodywork 2019;12(3):9–15.

16. Field T, Hernandez-Reif M, Diego M, et al. Cortisol decreases and serotonin and dopamine increase following massage therapy. Int J Neurosci 2005;115(10):1397–413.

17. Ferrell-Torry AT, Glick OJ. The use of therapeutic massage as a nursing intervention to modify anxiety and the perception of cancer pain. Cancer Nurs 1993;162:93–101.

18. Furlan AD, Giraldo M, Baskwill A, et al. Massage for low-back pain. Cochrane Database Syst Rev 2015;9:CD001929.

19. Miake-Lye IM, Mak S, Lee J, et al. Massage for pain: an evidence map. J Altern Complement Med 2019;25(5):475–502.

20. Niazi AK, Niazi SK. Mindfulness-based stress reduction: a non-pharmacological approach for chronic illnesses. N Am J Med Sci 2011;3(1):20–3.

21. Institute for Mindfulness-Based Approaches. What is MBSR?. Available at: https://www.institute-for-mindfulness.org/offer/mbsr/what-is-mbsr. Accessed Oct 26 2021.

22. Turner JA, Anderson ML, Balderson BH, et al. Mindfulness-based stress reduction and cognitive behavioral therapy for chronic low back pain: similar effects on mindfulness, catastrophizing, self-efficacy, and acceptance in a randomized controlled trial. Pain 2016;157(11):2434–44.
23. Available at: https://www.cms.gov/medicare-coverage-database/view/ncacal-decision-memo.aspx?proposed=N&NCAId=295. Accessed Oct 30 2021.
24. Chou R, Deyo R, Friedly J, et al. Noninvasive treatments for low back pain. Comparative Effectiveness review No. 169. Rockville, MD: Agency for Healthcare Research and Quality; 2016 (Prepared by the Pacific Northwest Evidence-based Practice Center under Contract No. 290-2012-00014-I.) AHRQ Publication No. 16-EHC004-EF. http://www.effectivehealthcare.ahrq.gov/reports/final.cfm.
25. Chou R, Deyo R, Friedly J, et al. Nonpharmacologic Therapies for Low Back Pain: A Systematic Review for an American College of Physicians Clinical Practice Guideline. Ann Intern Med 2017;166(7):493–505.
26. Skelly AC, Chou R, Dettori JR, et al. Noninvasive nonpharmacological treatment for chronic pain: a systematic review. Comparative Effectiveness review No. 209. (Prepared by the Pacific Northwest evidence-based practice center under Contract No. 290-2015-00009-I.) AHRQ publication No 18- EHC013-EF. Rockville, MD: Agency for Healthcare Research and Quality; 2018.
27. Vickers AJ, Vertosick EA, Lewith G, et al. Acupuncture for Chronic Pain: Update of an Individual Patient Data Meta-Analysis. J Pain 2018;19(5):455–74.
28. Xiang Y, He J, Li R. Appropriateness of sham or placebo acupuncture for randomized controlled trials of acupuncture for nonspecific low back pain: a systematic review and meta-analysis. J Pain Res 2018;(11):83–94.
29. Zeng Y, Chung JW. Acupuncture for chronic nonspecific low back pain: An overview of systematic reviews. Eur J Integr Med 2015;7(2):94–107.
30. American chronic pain association Resource Guide to chronic pain management, an integrated Guide to medical, interventional, Behavioral pharmacologic and Rehabilitation therapies. Feinberg S (ed.) American chronic pain association Inc., Rocklin, California. 2019. Available at: https://www.theacpa.org/wp-content/uploads/2019/02/ACPA_Resource_Guide_2019.pdf. Accessed May 13, 2019.
31. VA/DoD Clinical Practice Guideline for Diagnosis and Treatment of Low Back Pain. Department of Veterans Affairs, Department of Defense. Version 2.0 – 2017. Available at: https://www.healthquality.va.gov/guidelines/Pain/lbp/VADoDLBPCPG092917.pdf. Accessed October 29 2021
32. Mu J, Furlan AD, Lam WY, et al. Acupuncture for chronic nonspecific low back pain. Cochrane Database Syst Rev 2020;12(12):CD013814.
33. Moura CC, Chaves ECL, Cardoso ACLR, et al. Auricular acupuncture for chronic back pain in adults: a systematic review and metanalysis. Acupuntura auricular para dor crônica nas costas em adultos: revisão sistemática e metanálise. Rev Esc Enferm USP 2019;53:e03461.
34. Available at: https://clinicaltrials.gov/ct2/results?cond=Chronic+Pain&term=acupuncture&cntry=&state=&city=&dist.
35. Wong JJ, Côté P, Sutton DA, et al. Clinical practice guidelines for the noninvasive management of low back pain: A systematic review by the Ontario Protocol for Traffic Injury Management (OPTIMa) Collaboration. Eur J Pain 2017;21(2):201–16.
36. Godley E, Smith MA. Efficacy of acupressure for chronic low back pain: A systematic review. Complement Ther Clin Pract 2020;39:101146.

37. Yeganeh M, Baradaran HR, Qorbani M, et al. The effectiveness of acupuncture, acupressure and chiropractic interventions on treatment of chronic nonspecific low back pain in Iran: A systematic review and meta-analysis. Complement Ther Clin Pract 2017;27:11–8.

38. Murphy SL, Harris RE, Keshavarzi NR, et al. Self-Administered Acupressure for Chronic Low Back Pain: A Randomized Controlled Pilot Trial. Pain Med 2019; 20(12):2588–97.

39. Hsieh LL, Kuo C, Lee LH, et al. Treatment of low back pain by acupressure and physical therapy: randomised controlled trial. BMJ 2006;332:696–700.

40. Yang LH, Duan PB, Hou QM, et al. Efficacy of Auricular Acupressure for Chronic Low Back Pain: A Systematic Review and Meta-Analysis of Randomized Controlled Trials. Evid Based Complement Alternat Med 2017;2017:6383649.

41. Cherkin DC, Sherman KJ, Balderson BH, et al. Effect of mindfulness-based stress reduction vs cognitive behavioral therapy or usual care on back pain and functional limitations in adults with chronic low back pain: a randomized clinical trial. JAMA 2016;315:1240–9.

42. Krøll LS, Callesen HE, Carlsen LN, et al. Manual joint mobilisation techniques, supervised physical activity, psychological treatment, acupuncture and patient education for patients with tension-type headache. A systematic review and meta-analysis. J Headache Pain 2021;22(1):96.

43. Gildir S, Tüzün EH, Eroğlu G, et al. A randomized trial of trigger point dry needling versus sham needling for chronic tension-type headache. Medicine (Baltimore) 2019;98(8):e14520.

44. Murakami M, Fox L, Dijkers MP. Ear Acupuncture for Immediate Pain Relief-A Systematic Review and Meta-Analysis of Randomized Controlled Trials. Pain Med 2017;18(3):551–64.

45. Linde K, Allais G, Brinkhaus B, et al. Acupuncture for the prevention of episodic migraine. Cochrane Database Syst Rev 2016;2016(6):CD001218.

46. Deare JC, Zheng Z, Xue CC, et al. Acupuncture for treating fibromyalgia. Cochrane Database Syst Rev 2013;2013(5):CD007070.

47. Karatay S, Okur SC, Uzkeser H, et al. Effects of Acupuncture Treatment on Fibromyalgia Symptoms, Serotonin, and Substance P Levels: A Randomized Sham and Placebo-Controlled Clinical Trial. Pain Med 2018;19(3):615–28.

48. Asssefi NP, Sherman KJ, Jacobsen C, et al. A randomized clinical trial of acupuncture compared with sham acupuncture in fibromyalgia. Ann Intern Med 2005;143(1):10–9.

49. Martin DP, Sletten CD, Williams BA, et al. Improvement in fibromyalgia symptoms with acupuncture: results of a randomized controlled trial. Mayo Clin Proc 2006; 81(6):749–57.

50. Cao H, Li X, Han M, et al. Acupoint stimulation for fibromyalgia: a systematic review of randomized controlled trials. Evid Based Complement Alternat Med 2013; 2013:362831.

51. Skelly AC, Chou R, Dettori JR, et al. Noninvasive nonpharmacological treatment for chronic pain: a systematic review update. Rockville (MD): Agency for Healthcare Research and Quality (US); 2020. Report No.: 20-EHC009.

52. Kaplan KH, Goldenberg DL, Nadeau MG. The impact of a meditation-based stress reduction program on fibromyalgia. Gen Hosp Psychiatry 1993;15(5): 284–9.

53. Kolasinski SL, Neogi T, Hochberg MC, et al. 2019 American College of Rheumatology/Arthritis Foundation Guideline for the Management of Osteoarthritis of the

Hand, Hip, and Knee [published correction appears in Arthritis Care Res (Hoboken). 2021 May;73(5):764. Arthritis Care Res (Hoboken) 2020;72(2):149–62.

54. Manheimer E, Cheng K, Linde K, et al. Acupuncture for peripheral joint osteoarthritis. Cochrane Database Syst Rev 2010;1:CD001977.
55. Hinman RS, McCrory P, Pirotta M, et al. Acupuncture for chronic knee pain: a randomized clinical trial. JAMA 2014;312(13):1313–22.
56. Chen LX, Mao JJ, Fernandes S, et al. Integrating acupuncture with exercise-based physical therapy for knee osteoarthritis: a randomized controlled trial. J Clin Rheumatol 2013;19(6):308–16.
57. Tu JF, Yang JW, Shi GX, et al. Efficacy of Intensive Acupuncture Versus Sham Acupuncture in Knee Osteoarthritis: A Randomized Controlled Trial. Arthritis Rheum 2021;73(3):448–58.
58. Dunning J, Butts R, Young I, et al. Periosteal Electrical Dry Needling as an Adjunct to Exercise and Manual Therapy for Knee Osteoarthritis: A Multicenter Randomized Clinical Trial. Clin J Pain 2018;34(12):1149–58.
59. Li LW, Harris RE, Tsodikov A, et al. Self-acupressure for older adults with symptomatic knee osteoarthritis: a randomized controlled trial. Arthritis Care Res (Hoboken) 2018;70(2):221–9.
60. Nelson NL, Churilla JR. Massage therapy for pain and function in patients with arthritis: a systematic review of randomized controlled trials. Am J Phys Med Rehabil 2017;96(9):665–72.
61. Perlman AI, Ali A, Njike VY, et al. Massage therapy for osteoarthritis of the knee: a randomized dose-finding trial. PLoS ONE [Electronic Resource] 2012;7(2):e30248.
62. Shetty GB, Shetty B, Mooventhan A. Efficacy of Acupuncture in the Management of Primary Dysmenorrhea: A Randomized Controlled Trial. J Acupunct Meridian Stud 2018;11(4):153–8.
63. Falk J, Thomas B, Kirkwood J, et al. PEER systematic review of randomized controlled trials: Management of chronic neuropathic pain in primary care. Can Fam Physician 2021;67(5):e130–40.
64. Available at: https://www.acupuncturetoday.com/schools/Accessed 30 Oct 2021
65. You J, Li H, Xie D, et al. Acupuncture for Chronic Pain-Related Depression: A Systematic Review and Meta-Analysis. Pain Res Manag 2021;2021:6617075.
66. Fan AY, Stumpf SH, Faggert Alemi S, et al. Distribution of licensed acupuncturists and educational institutions in the United States at the start of 2018. Complement Ther Med 2018;41:295–301.

# Systems-Based Practice in Chronic Pain Management

Margot Latrese Savoy, MD, MPH, FABC, CPE[a,b,*]

## KEYWORDS

- Practice management • Chronic pain • Systems-based practice • Primary care
- Pain management

## KEY POINTS

- Care for patients with chronic pain is a complex task requiring coordination between a wide range of systems each with their own policies and procedures.
- Systems engineering concepts and models are useful tools to apply when managing complex systems within systems such as chronic pain management.
- Systems-based practice, a core ACGME competency, requires residents to develop awareness of and responsiveness to the larger context and system of health care and the ability to call on system resources effectively to provide care that is of optimal value.

## INTRODUCTION

Chronic pain is a significant public health concern in the United States impacting between 11% and 40% of Americans.[1] In addition to being one of the most common reasons for seeing medical care, chronic pain is linked to loss of mobility, reduction of daily activities, reduced quality of life, worsening mental health including increased rates of depression and anxiety, and increased dependence on opioids.[2–5] Chronic pain contributes to an estimated $560 billion each year in direct medical costs, lost productivity, and disability programs.[1]

As we work to reign in the markedly growing cost of health care and disability in the United States, a new appreciation of manufacturing and engineering design and concepts has emerged. Interest in applying these tools, known to be valuable for improving the delivery and reducing the cost of manufacturing and business practices, in medical care has blossomed.

The Toyota Production System, referred to as lean or just-in-time thinking, leverages intentionally focusing on waste elimination as a way to achieve optimal

[a] American Academy of Family Physicians, 1133 Connecticut Ave, NW Suite 1100 Washington, DC 20036, USA; [b] Family & Community Medicine and Urban Bioethics & Population Health, Lewis Katz School of Medicine at Temple University, Philadelphia, PA, USA
* 5278 Winter View Drive, Alexandria, VA 22312.
*E-mail address:* Margot.Savoy@tuhs.temple.edu
Twitter: @MargotSavoy (M.L.S.)

Prim Care Clin Office Pract 49 (2022) 485–496
https://doi.org/10.1016/j.pop.2022.01.004
primarycare.theclinics.com
0095-4543/22/© 2022 Elsevier Inc. All rights reserved.

efficiency. Motorola refined a Six Sigma strategy that seeks defects and viability in processes though statistics data that can be removed leading to optimally improved overall quality. Combined processes called "Lean Six Sigma" have successfully been applied to the health care industry in manufacturing, patient care delivery, and business processes. Similarly applying systems engineering concepts to medicine opens the door to addressing a wide range of performance gaps through a structured, evidence-based approach.

## HEALTH CARE AS SYSTEM

Merriam Webster defines a system as a regularly interacting or interdependent group of items forming a unified whole.[6] Put another way, a system is a collection of independent things or elements that when connected together form a particular output or outcome. Consider a typical primary care practice. The practice is made up of individuals who are each independent roles or people yet work together to create the practice experience.

### The Patient-Centered Medical Home

A primary care practice is a carefully curated system that engages several valuable team members and services to deliver patient-centered care. The Patient-Centered Medical Home (PCMH) model implemented widely in the United States organizes this system of primary care delivery.[7] Defined by the Agency for Healthcare Quality and Research, a PCMH is "not simply as a place but as a model of the organization of primary care that delivers the core functions of primary health care" as noted in **Table 1**.

**Fig. 1** demonstrates a primary care office setting as an example of a system. Although some of these positions or roles may not be embedded within all primary care practices, it is easy to see how different roles intersect from scheduling the appointment to rooming the patient to diagnosing and treating the patient through supporting the patient to create a system that delivers on the desires outcome.

### The Medical Neighborhood

The PCMH is inadequate to meet all of a patient's care needs. Attempting to capture the larger complexity of delivering primary care by leveraging community resources that partner with health care services is known as the medical neighborhood. Some define the neighborhood as the addition of specialty providers, hospitals, and other clinicians working in partnership with primary care to provide complete and coordinated care; this notably overlooks the community-based services that may be independent of the medical system, which are also key contributors to the patient's medical care. In this broader definition, the medical neighbors shown in **Fig. 2** include both nonclinical partners like community centers, faith-based organizations, schools, employers, public health agencies, YMCAs, Meals on Wheels, and additional clinical partners such as home health, long-term care, and other clinical providers.[8,9]

### Health Care as a Systems of Systems

The medical neighborhood is a useful framework, yet it still fails to capture the incredible complexity of the US Healthcare system. A better depiction is the concept known as systems of systems (SoS) in which multiple, dispersed, independent systems are viewed in context as part of a larger, more complex system.[10] A simplified depiction highlighting the multiple intersecting systems is seen in **Fig. 3**. Patients with medical

| Table 1 Agency for healthcare quality and research core function of a patient-centered medical home | |
|---|---|
| Comprehensive care | • Accountable for meeting the large majority of each patient's physical and mental health care needs, including prevention and wellness, acute care, and chronic care<br>• Leverages a multidisciplinary team of care providers and clinicians<br>• May form virtual connections between smaller practices to expand access for a community |
| Patient centered | • Relationship based<br>• Orientation to the whole person<br>• Respectful of each patient's unique needs, culture, values, and preferences<br>• Recognizes patients and families as core team members |
| Coordinated care | • Coordinates care across all elements of the broader health care system, including specialty care, hospitals, home health care, and community services and supports |
| Accessible services | • Responsive to patient needs and preferences through shorter waiting times for urgent needs, enhanced in-person hours, around-the-clock telephone or electronic access to a member of the care team, and alternative methods of communication |
| Quality & safety | • Ongoing engagement in activities such as using evidence-based medicine and clinical decision-support tools to guide shared decision making with patients and families, engaging in performance measurement and improvement, measuring and responding to patient experiences and patient satisfaction, and practicing population health management |

*Data from* Defining patient centered medical home. Agency for Healthcare Research and Quality. Available at: https://pcmh.ahrq.gov/page/defining-pcmh. Accessed November 21, 2021.

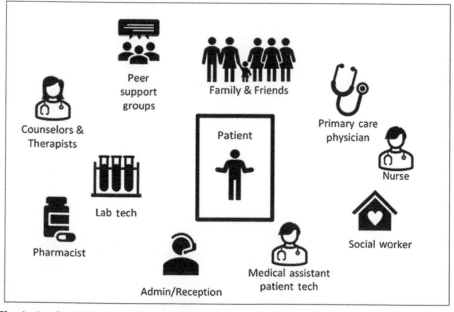

**Fig. 1.** A primary care practice's system.

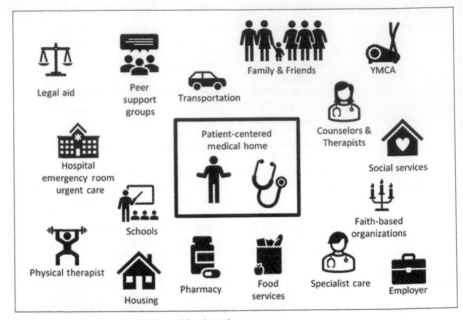

**Fig. 2.** Example of a medical neighborhood.

illness can find themselves wandering throughout this complex maze of systems each with their own policies, procedures, and processes attempting to receive care. Patients experiencing chronic pain frequently find themselves in this position. To improve the patient's experience, care, and outcomes, the medical system can leverage system engineering principles.

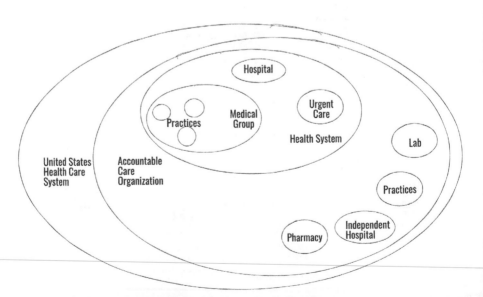

**Fig. 3.** A simplified example of a health care system of systems.

## SYSTEMS ENGINEERING

Modern systems engineering is defined as the discipline "which concentrates on the design and application of the whole as distinct from the parts, looking at a problem in its entirety, taking account of all the facets and the variables and linking the social to the technological."[11] Health care systems engineering is a subset that takes into account the complex service delivery and mixed outcomes that are unique to health care delivery.

When applied to the US health system, a complex system composed of smaller complex systems, systems engineering allows us to view individual processes as opportunities for improvement as well as the intersections between systems and the functioning of the overall system. The National Academies of Medicine define a systems approach to health as "one that applies scientific insights to understand the elements that influence health outcomes; models the relationships between those elements; and alters design, processes, or policies based on the resultant knowledge in order to produce better health at lower cost."[12]

To optimize health care outcomes, typically health system engineers will leverage aspects of operations research and analytics with human factors engineering. Operations research and analytics uses algorithms, modeling and simulations to identify problems and test solutions to complex problems. Human factors engineering is the application of human factors information to the design of tools, machines, systems, tasks, jobs, and environments for safe, comfortable, and effective human use. Human factors refer to environmental, organizational, and job factors and human and individual characteristics, which influence behavior at work in a way that can affect health and safety.[10]

The health care systems engineer's toolbox contains several resources that are well known to physicians through increased focus in recent years on quality improvement and safety training. Overall the broad stages described by the National Academies of Medicine (**Box 1**) are used; they align easily with the successful and well-known Plan-Do-See-Act model most clinicians have been exposed to. Examples of common tools or techniques used in the various stages are included in **Table 2**.

If health care leaders or practicing clinicians in the various interconnected medical systems are unaware of the intricacies of the larger system, improvements made in one area will not successfully spread across the wider system and in the worst case, could create new and worsening challenges or obstacles for the patients trying to navigate their care. To address the need for this foundational critical awareness, graduate medical education has incorporated systems-based practice as a core competency for all physicians.

## SYSTEMS-BASED PRACTICE

The Accreditation Council for Graduate Medical Education defines systems-based practice as "awareness of and responsiveness to the larger context and system of health care and the ability to call on system resources effectively to provide care that is of optimal value."[13] Reframed another way, it is ensuring that physicians have the knowledge and skills (**Box 2**) needed to identify resources outside of the 4 walls of their practice that can improve the care they deliver to their patients. Successful implementation of systems-based practice includes effectively incorporating interprofessional teamwork, community resources, team-based care, patient safety, hospital readmissions, use of evidence-based medicine, transitions of care, and care for the underserved, including social determinants of health into the routine delivery of health care services.[14]

> **Box 1**
> **National Academies of Medicine stages in systems approach to health care**
>
> 1. *Identification:* Identify the multiple elements involved in caring for patients and promoting the health of individuals and populations.
>
> 2. *Description:* Describe how those elements operate independently and interdependently.
>
> 3. *Alteration:* Change the design of organizations, processes, or policies to enhance the results of the interplay and engage in a continuous improvement process that promotes learning at all levels.
>
> 4. *Implementation:* Operationalize the integration of the new dynamics to facilitate the ways people, processes, facilities, equipment, and organizations all work together to achieve better care at lower cost.
>
> *From* Kaplan, G., G. Bo-Linn, P. Carayon, P. Pronovost, W. Rouse, P. Reid, and R. Saunders. 2013. Bringing a Systems Approach to Health. NAM Perspectives. Discussion Paper, National Academy of Medicine, Washington, DC. Accessed 11-28-2021. https://nam.edu/perspectives-2013-bringing-a-systems-approach-to-health/.

Although this complex arrangement of interconnecting systems is a convenient way to organize the health care system as we seek opportunities to improve it, from the patient perspective the view is notably different. A patient's journey or experience may interact with multiple aspects of the system, but often their encounters are disjointed, frustrating, and lead to delays in the outcomes most important to them— relief from their illness, management of their symptoms, or cure from their condition.

**Table 2**
**Examples of health care system engineering tools**

| | |
|---|---|
| Definition of the problem | • Define the boundaries and scope of the problem<br>• Stakeholder identification and management<br>• Lifecycle mapping<br>• Value stream process mapping<br>• SWOT analysis (operational deficiencies and technological opportunities)<br>• Workflow/usability analysis<br>• Observation research<br>• Root cause analysis (fishbone diagrams, 5 whys) |
| Investigate alternatives | • Decision trees<br>• Trade-off analysis<br>• Risk management |
| Develop the solution | • Concept development<br>• Functional analysis<br>• Modeling potential outcomes<br>• Implementation design<br>• Process redesign techniques (Lean Six Sigma)<br>• Agile /Lean development principles |
| Launch and assess the solution | • Organizational change management<br>• Spiral, Agile, and Lean Startup delivery practices<br>• Metrics and benchmarking |

*Data from* Kaplan, G., G. Bo-Linn, P. Carayon, P. Pronovost, W. Rouse, P. Reid, and R. Saunders. 2013. Bringing a Systems Approach to Health. NAM Perspectives. Discussion Paper, National Academy of Medicine, Washington, DC. Accessed 11-28-2021. https://nam.edu/perspectives-2013-bringing-a-systems-approach-to-health/. Accessed 11-28-2021.

---

**Box 2**
**Key skills, activities, and components of systems-based practice**

- Work effectively in various health care delivery settings and systems relevant to their clinical specialty.

- Coordinate patient care within the health care system relevant to their clinical specialty.

- Incorporate considerations of cost awareness and risk-benefit analysis in patient care.

- Advocate for quality patient care and optimal patient care systems.

- Work in interprofessional teams to enhance patient safety and improve patient care quality.

- Participate in identifying system errors and in implementing potential systems solutions.

*Key Components:*
- Knowledge of the larger context and system of health care
- Use of resources within the system to provide excellent patient care
- Knowledge of patient safety and advocacy

*Data from* Moskowitz EJ, Nash DB. ACGME competencies: practice-based learning and systems-based practice. Am J Med Qual. 2007;22:351–382.

---

**Fig. 4** demonstrates a patient's journey through the health care system while experiencing chronic back pain. Throughout the journey clinicians and practices may have appropriately applied evidence-based medicine and best practices such as early referral to physical therapy or minimizing delays in handoff from inpatient care back to primary care. However, the overall system still failed to deliver satisfactory outcomes for the patient, and without intentionally taking a larger systems-based approach, additional quality improvements seeking to aid the patient ultimately exacerbate the disparity between the high-quality and efficient system by the physician's measures and the patient's experience with ongoing pain, disability, and inability to earn a living.

## CASE STUDY: STARTING A NEW PRIMARY CARE PAIN MANAGEMENT PRACTICE
### Case Presentation

You are the medical director at a large family medicine practice. Recently you hired 3 new physicians to join your group and you are meeting with them this morning to prepare for their start dates. One of the new physicians reminds you that she cares for several patients with chronic pain and prescribes medication-assisted treatment for opiate use disorder. The 2 other doctors immediately lit up excited to share that they too included chronic pain management in their practices. As they started to talk among themselves about the processes, policies, and staff training they would need now as they joined your practices your heart sank a bit.

### Case Questions

- You had been excited to offer the new service to the community, but now you are unsure where to start—what does a practice need to set up to be successful?
- Are there best practices for organizing chronic pain care within a primary care practice?
- How do we create a practice culture that makes our new physicians feel welcome and the patients feel they are in a safe place for care?
- Where can we find resources to get this process started?

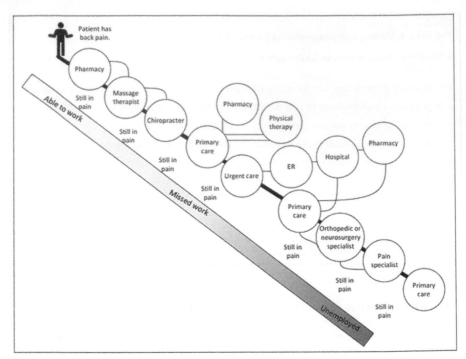

**Fig. 4.** A patient's back pain patient journey.

### Case Discussion: Improving Chronic Pain Management Using a Systems-Based Approach

You correctly identify chronic pain management as an example of a medical SoS, which means you will need to take care not only to develop the proper approaches within your practice but also how your practice will connect to resources within your community. After some research you decide to use the National Academies of Medicine stages (see **Box 1**) to approach your system change.

### IDENTIFICATION

You decide to convene a working group to think collectively through how to best stand up the chronic pain services. Thinking through the guest list for the initial meeting you decide to extend invitations not only to your interested physicians but also to include any interested clinicians/staff in the practice and members of your patient-family advisory council. As you begin thinking about who else should attend, you begin to focus on who are your key stakeholders.[9]

Applying 5 questions (**Box 3**)[15] you narrow down the list to the top organizations your practice refers patients with chronic pain to, including the local physical therapist, the medical legal aid group that assists patients with disability rights and benefits, a pharmacist at the outpatient pharmacy of the local hospital where many of your patients have their prescriptions filled, and the social worker at the emergency room where patients present after hours for pain relief.

While organizing the meeting agenda you quickly determine that the first meetings should not be for decision making but rather should be used as listening sessions and process clarification. You use the meeting to hear about what the experience is in your

> **Box 3**
> **Applying five questions to identify key stakeholders**
>
> - Does the stakeholder have a fundamental impact on your organization's performance?
> - Can you clearly identify what you want from the stakeholder?
> - Is the relationship dynamic—that is, do you want it to grow?
> - Can you exist without or easily replace the stakeholder?
> - Has the stakeholder already been identified through another relationship?
>
> *Data from* Graham K. Five questions to identify key stakeholders. Harvard Business Review. 2014. Accessed 11-21-2021. https://hbr.org/2014/03/five-questions-to-identify-key-stakeholders.

practice both for the patient and the clinicians/staff uncovering not only barriers to care but also additional community partners to engage such as the local chronic pain peer support group. Over the next few meetings the team works together to outline the strengths, weaknesses, opportunities, and threats of your current approach to chronic pain. In addition, you develop a process map that outlines a patient's journey when presenting with chronic care. Deeper dives on critical steps in the plan were explored by asking why we are doing it this way multiple times to get to the root of the issues.

## DESCRIPTION

Additional meetings including stakeholders in your local health system and community partners allow your workgroup to develop a clearer picture of how various external systems of chronic pain management care are interwoven. After agreeing on the state of the current system, the work group uses decision trees to begin prioritizing which barriers are most critical to address first. Staring down a long list of possible projects, your team ultimately opts to focus on the policies and processes within your control as a starting place while recognizing that advocating for changes in other systems will continue to be needed to achieve optimal outcomes. Specifically, they hone in on the start of the process—how do you even know a patient has chronic pain and what assessment should be used?

## ALTERATION

Because the workgroup identifies a lack of clarity about pain management and what the evidence-based guidelines are, your team decides to choose an evidence-based guideline to implement and help drive the practice's policy and process changes. Your research uncovers several valuable resources. Combining the American Academy of Family Physician's Chronic Pain Management toolkit (https://www.aafp.org/family-physician/patient-care/care-resources/pain-management/aafp-chronic-pain-management-toolkit.html), the Centers for Disease Control and Prevention's Opioid Prescribing Guideline Resources (https://www.cdc.gov/opioids/providers/prescribing/index.html), and the National Academy of Medicine's First, Do No Harm: Marshaling Clinician Leadership to Counter the Opioid Epidemic (https://nam.edu/first-no-harm-nam-special-publication/), your team has access to up-to-date evidence-based tools that address specific gaps in the practice flow, standardize evaluation and treatment, discuss pain management goals, and identify at-risk patients.

## IMPLEMENTATION

Using a Plan-Do-See-Act approach your team launches a series of quality improvements, starting with educating the practice team about their identified gaps in knowledge around chronic pain and substance use disorder and then tackling their trauma-informed care and diversity and inclusion trainings to help them mitigate the stigma of chronic pain when patients are receiving care in the practice. The team develops a dashboard of key indicators that will be their guide to tracking progress as they continue to improve care. After clarifying the optimal process and tools using a paper system, they are built into accessible workflows within the electronic medical record. Ongoing patient input highlights glitches and unforeseen barriers that are addressed by the working group. As the patient volume increases, you begin to encourage members of your frequent referral sites to become more active in the working group optimizing referrals and patient experience across handoffs.

## SUMMARY

Chronic pain management in the primary care setting can feel overwhelming; it is a complex system of systems and dynamic processes that make accessing care difficult for patients. Systems-based approaches allow clinical teams to identify opportunities efficiently and effectively for removing barriers, fixing broken processes, and redesigning a care pathway that optimizes best evidence, improves patient outcomes, and saves money.

## CLINICS CARE POINTS

- Use system-based tools (eg, Strengths-Weaknesses-Opportunties-Threats [SWOT], Plan-Do-See-Act [PDSA]) to identify opportunities for improvement, develop and implement solutions, and monitor progress.
- Include patients living with chronic pain and a wide range of community program representatives in your chronic pain management program development.
- Seek sustainable solutions to address barriers to evidence-based chronic pain management rather than workarounds.
- When developing your practice approach to chronic pain use evidence-based guides and resources such as American Academy of Family Physician's Chronic Pain Management toolkit (https://www.aafp.org/family-physician/patient-care/care-resources/pain-management/aafp-chronic-pain-management-toolkit.html), the Centers for Disease Control and Prevention's Opioid Prescribing Guideline Resources (https://www.cdc.gov/opioids/providers/prescribing/index.html), and the National Academy of Medicine's First, Do No Harm: Marshaling Clinician Leadership to Counter the Opioid Epidemic (https://nam.edu/first-no-harm-nam-special-publication/).

## DISCLOSURE

The author has no financial conflicts to disclose.

## REFERENCES

1. Interagency Pain Research Coordinating Committee. National pain strategy: a Comprehensive population health-level strategy for pain. Washington, DC: US Department of Health and Human Services, National Institutes of Health; 2016.

2. Schappert SM, Burt CW. Ambulatory care visits to physician offices, hospital outpatient departments, and emergency departments: United States, 2001–02. Vital Health Stat 2006;13:1–66.

3. Gureje O, Von Korff M, Simon GE, et al. Persistent pain and well-being. A World Health Organization study in primary care. JAMA 1998;280:147–51.

4. Smith BH, Elliott AM, Chambers WA, et al. The impact of chronic pain in the community. Fam Pract 2001;18:292–9.

5. Institute of Medicine. Relieving pain in America: a blueprint for transforming prevention, care, education, and research. Washington, DC: National Academies Press; 2011.

6. "system." Merriam-Webster.com. Merriam-Webster. 2021. Available at: https://www.merriam-webster.com/dictionary/system. Accessed November 20 2021.

7. Defining patient centered medical home. Agency for Healthcare Research and Quality. Available at: https://pcmh.ahrq.gov/page/defining-pcmh. Accessed November 21 2021.

8. Patient Centered Primary Care Collaborative. Med Neighborhood 2021. Available at: https://www.pcpcc.org/content/medical-neighborhood. Accessed November 28 2021.

9. Taylor EF, Lake T, Nysenbaum J, et al. Coordinating care in the medical neighborhood: critical components and available mechanisms. Rockville, MD: Agency for Healthcare Research and Quality; 2011. White Paper (Prepared by Mathematica Policy Research under Contract No. HHSA290200900019I TO2). AHRQ Publication No. 11-0064.

10. Gosbee J. Human factors engineering and patient safety. Qual Saf Health Care 2002;11:352–4.

11. The Defence Engineering Group. Conquering Complexity: Lessons in Defence Systems Acquisition. University College London. 2005.

12. Compton WD, Fanjiang G, Grossman JH, et al. Building a better delivery system: a new engineering/health care partnership. Washington DC: National Academies Press; 2005. Available at: https://nam.edu/perspectives-2013-bringing-a-systems-approach-to-health/. Accessed November 28 2021.

13. NEJM Knowledge+ Team. Exploring the ACGME core competencies: systems-based practice 2016. Available at: https://knowledgeplus.nejm.org/blog/acgme-core-competencies-systems-based-practice/. Accessed September 21 2021.

14. Moskowitz EJ, Nash DB. ACGME competencies: Practice-based learning and systems-based practice. Am J Med Qual 2007;22:351–82.

15. Graham K. Five Questions to Identify Key Stakeholders. Harv Business Rev 2014. Available at: https://hbr.org/2014/03/five-questions-to-identify-key-stakeholders. Accessed November 21 2021.

## FURTHER READINGS

Available at: https://www.aafp.org/family-physician/patient-care/care-resources/pain-management/aafp-chronic-pain-management-toolkit.html

Available at: https://www.ncbi.nlm.nih.gov/books/NBK43731/

Available at: https://www.aafp.org/afp/2002/0701/p36.html

Available at: https://www.practicalpainmanagement.com/resources/practice-management/chronic-pain-program-primary-care-setting

Allen E, Zerzan J, Choo C, et al. Teaching Systems-Based Practice to Residents by Using Independent Study Projects. Acad Med 2005;80(2):125–8.

Duffy D, Cable C. Teaching Systems-Based Practice. which can be found by following the link at. Available at: http://www.hematology.org/Training/Directors/4699.aspx.

Dyne PL, et al. Systems-Based Practice: The Sixth Core Competency. Acad Emer Med 2002;9:1270–7.

Johnson JK, Miller SH, Horowitz SD. Systems-Based Practice: Improving the Safety and Quality of Patient Care by Recognizing and Improving the Systems in Which We Work. In: Henriksen K, Battles JB, Keyes MA, Grady ML, editors. Advances in Patient Safety: New Directions and Alternative Approaches (Vol. 2: Culture and Redesign). Rockville (MD): Agency for Healthcare Research and Quality; 2008.

Kerfoot BP, Conlin PR, Travison T, et al. Web-Based Education in Systems-Based Practice: A Randomized Trial. Arch Intern Med 2007;167:361–6.

Nabors C, Peterson SJ, Weems R, et al. A Multidisciplinary Approach for Teaching Systems-based Practice to Internal Medicine Residents. J Grad Med Educ 2011;3(1):75–80.

Tomolo A, Caron A, Perz ML, et al. The outcomes card. Development of a systems-based practice educational tool. J Gen Intern Med 2005;20:769–71.

# Ethical Challenges in Chronic Pain

Kathleen Reeves, MD*, Nora Jones, PhD

## KEYWORDS

- Ethics • Chronic pain • Urban bioethics • Agency • Social justice • Solidarity

## KEY POINTS

- Current bioethics principles fail to provide an adequate toolbox for clinicians to be sure they are providing the most ethical care for patients suffering from chronic pain.
- Adding the urban bioethics principles of agency, social justice, and solidarity will greatly enhance a provider's ability to engage in ethical care with patients suffering from chronic pain.
- Medical education needs to include curricula around agency, social justice, and solidarity for future physicians to be sure physicians are well trained to provide ethical care in the management of chronic pain.

## INTRODUCTION

The ethical obligation to treat pain is recognized by most major health care professional organizations, including the World Health Organization, the American Medical Association, the American Nursing Association, the American Academy of Pediatrics, and the Agency for Health Care Policy and Research.[1] We know that even though chronic pain is more prevalent in the US population than diabetes, heart disease, and cancer combined, the health care system in the United States has failed to effectively treat the epidemic of chronic pain.[2] Medicine has many of the answers to evidence-based, effective treatment of chronic pain. Where medicine has failed is in not assuring these treatment modalities are applied equitably and ethically for all patients. Although this disconnect has many sources, our focus here is on the role bioethics may have played in the problem—and how it can, with some important modifications, contribute to the solution.

Pain is one of the more complicated conditions providers face. In addition to any clinical doubt that might arise when subjective accounts of pain cannot be supported by objective measures, the contemporary management of pain involves other forms of doubt. Managing pain involves navigating questions of addiction and stigma, the role

Department of Urban Health and Population Science, Center for Urban Bioethics, Lewis Katz School of Medicine at Temple University, Kresge Hall Suite 320, 3220 North Broad Street, Philadelphia, PA 19140, USA
* Corresponding author.
E-mail address: kreeves@temple.edu

Prim Care Clin Office Pract 49 (2022) 497–506
https://doi.org/10.1016/j.pop.2022.01.002

of profit in health care, and the identity of clinicians. We believe our work within the expanding field of urban bioethics provides a framework for understanding the variety of implicated stakeholders along with their social contexts and can be used to chart a pragmatic path forward toward more ethical and effective clinical management of pain.

## Bioethics and the Management of Pain

Bioethics is a field of study that contributes codes for naming right versus wrong actions and a toolbox to help make a choice when faced with multiple "rights." Bioethics provides various theories that can lead to developing a roadmap that help direct choice, develop policy, and affect care delivery. Deontology, or following one's duty, and Consequentialism, maximizing the "good," are both problematic when it comes to supporting the treatment of chronic pain. Deontology creates too narrow a view to include all stakeholders and Consequentialism does not allow for a unified approach by all the varying stakeholders involved in the treatment of chronic pain.

Principlism is the bioethics toolbox most commonly applied to the treatment of pain. It is grounded in the classic bioethics principles of autonomy, beneficence, nonmaleficence, and justice.[3] Autonomy, the right of an individual to determine what happens to their own body, is the principle of most importance to patients and their surrogates. Practicing with an eye to beneficence and nonmaleficence, in other words to prioritizing the "good" for the patient and avoiding harm, are principles most relevant to health care providers. Justice, most traditionally defined as the fair allocation of scarce resources, is a governing concern for health care institutions (**Fig. 1**). Although this framework may cover some aspects of the interaction between a patient and a provider in the treatment of pain, it does not fully consider the interplay between health systems, insurers, pharmaceutical companies, law enforcement, government, and societal norms.[4]

With this paper we would like to propose a different bioethics lens that provides a more effective toolbox for giving the practitioner and the patient greater capacity to realize health and health equity for patients and communities suffering from chronic pain. Urban bioethics is a field that was first described by Jeffery Blustein and Alan Fleischman in 2004.[5] Currently, the discipline of urban bioethics is being reclaimed with work in the Center for Urban Bioethics at the Lewis Katz School of Medicine at Temple University. This work has expanded on the work from Blustein and Fleischman as well as the basic bioethical principles described by Beauchamp and Childress to specifically address unique needs experienced by patients and populations in dense, diverse, and disparity-laden urban spaces.[3] Although addiction and the ethical

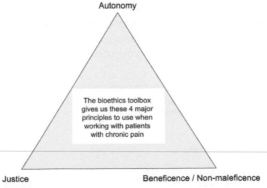

Fig. 1. The bioethics toolbox.

problem of pain management exists in all areas of the United States—rural, suburban, and urban—the additional urban bioethics principles provide a productive lens for rethinking our ethical approach to pain management.

Urban Bioethics centers on advocating for an expanded list of principles that includes agency, social justice, and solidarity. This set of principles, when used in conjunction with the capability theory of bioethics, provides a clearer map to create prevention and treatment plans that prioritize ethical practice and equity. The capability approach highlights 2 claims: first, the claim that the freedom, both positive and negative freedoms, to achieve well-being is of primary importance and, second, that well-being should be understood in terms of people's capabilities.[6] The only way to truly realize the capability theory is to have principles that take into account each person's context; the role culture, history, and society have played in that context; and a framework for solution that binds stakeholders together in a way that leads to a collective vision.

Our hope is to show how the application of traditional bioethics to the management of chronic pain is insufficient and even detrimental to achieving ethical, equitable care while exploring how this urban bioethics toolbox that can help create capacity for health equity in the care of patients suffering from chronic pain.

## DISCUSSION
### Autonomy Becomes Agency

Understanding and defining autonomy has long been a topic of discussion within bioethics. Autonomous choice, as defined by Beauchamp and Childress, involves analyzing an autonomous action in terms of, "normal choosers who act (i) intentionally, (ii) with understanding, and (iii) without controlling influences that determine their action."[3]

Grisso and Appelbaum's work regarding competence and consent as well as Jonsen, Siegler, and Winslade's writings in clinical ethics speak about the importance of self-determination and the promotion of well-being.[7,8] Jansen, Siegler, and Winslade defined autonomy in the clinical arena as follows in 1982:

> Patient preferences are ethically significant because they make explicit the values of self-determination and personal autonomy that are deeply rooted in the ethics of our culture. Autonomy is the moral right to choose and follow one's own plan of life and action.[8]

Autonomy defined as self-determination and self-governance assumes patient context plays little, if any, role in decision-making. The management of chronic pain requires a keen understanding of how a patient's context affects their ability to make a truly informed decision: to have competency. All patients do not respond in the same way to pain and to the medications that treat pain. An ethical response to the patient in pain requires an understanding of that patient's context and how this narrative affects their response to pain management. If a practitioner does not know how a patient's context affects their experience of pain and their experience of pain management, the patient cannot have access to what is needed to realize autonomy.

Knowing more about a patient's historical context will help a care giver provide more ethical care; this is particularly important regarding a history of childhood trauma; this is especially the case with the disease of chronic pain. The origin and evolution of attention to Adverse Childhood Experience (ACE) is an example of how an engaged approach to addressing an "epidemic" more evident in distressed communities can yield incredible insight and provide the necessary context of a patient's experience.

ACEs were first defined in the late 1990s by Felitti and associates based on their survey of middle-class adult patients in the Kaiser Permanente Health System in Southern California that correlated different types of stressful experiences in childhood with chronic disease and health outcomes later in life. With 2 waves of survey data covering more than 17,000 adults, these original ACE studies found that two-thirds of participants had exposure to at least 1 ACE, and 1 in 9 had an ACE score of 5 or more. In addition to revealing that ACEs were more common than many had expected, the study found a graded relationship between number of ACEs and chronic disease, including chronic pain syndrome.[9,10]

The import of these powerful results has limited generalizability in 2 respects, however. Demographically, the original ACEs studies surveyed primarily white, upper middle class, college educated, and insured individuals. Individuals living and working in more diverse urban environments also found that the ACEs from the original study did not address their neighborhood and community experiences that created significant sources of stress. This concern led to the development of the Urban ACE study in Philadelphia and follow-up studies in other urban spaces.[11,12] Through literature review as well as qualitative data from African American and Latino youth in Philadelphia, the themes of the expanded ACEs were developed to include factors related to social location, such as exposure to community violence, experiencing racism, living in an unsafe neighborhood, experiencing bullying, and having a history of living in foster care. The results of the Urban ACE study showed that the prevalence of the conventional ACEs was higher in the Philadelphia dataset compared with the original and most other subsequent studies: 72.9% of Philadelphians had at least 1 conventional ACE, 47.6% had 1 to 3 ACEs, and 20.7% were found to have an ACE score of 4 or more. For the 5 expanded ACEs, they found that 63.4% of the population surveyed had at least 1 exposure, 50% had a score of 1 to 3 ACEs, and 13.4% had 3 or more. A further analysis of the expanded ACEs found that 40.5% of participants had witnessed community violence, 34.5% experienced racial discrimination, and 27.3% felt their neighborhood was unsafe. The most distressed, urban neighborhoods in Philadelphia are in north Philadelphia, surrounding our health system, and ACE surveys from these communities reported that more than 48% of adults experienced 4 or more adverse childhood experiences. We know that such exposure to childhood adversity can increase the likelihood of a chronic pain syndrome and of a substance use disorder each by 7 times or more.[13]

*Agency* here refers first to a person's ability to see a complete range of options possible in a given situation and second, to the capacity to carry out a particular choice. Our agency depends on the experiences we have had, experiences influenced by our gender, sexual orientation, skin color, class background, educational experiences, schools attended—in other words, by our context. A bioethics that stops at respecting a patient's abstract autonomy, but does not account for their particular agency, pushes the ethical boundaries, and a clinician who focuses only on autonomy without attention to agency does a disservice to their patient. We are setting them up for failure if they cannot take our advice, wasting resources when they are readmitted for preventable recurrences of illness, and contributing to our own burnout by making the same mistakes again and again.

For a patient to have agency, this would require that the patient be made aware of the research around childhood adversity and chronic pain. The practitioner would also need to be up to date regarding how an awareness of this association can alter which options are provided to patient and these opportunities are explained. A commitment to agency over autonomy would require that medical education include this research around childhood adversity into its curricula and that there be an expectation that all patients suffering from chronic pain be adequately educated and evaluated regarding adverse childhood experiences and the associated ramifications (**Fig. 2**).

### Beneficence/Nonmaleficence Becomes Social Justice

Social justice requires equitable access to opportunity as well as an acknowledgment of both disparity and privilege. Beneficence and non-maleficence within bioethics are not concerned with equity but with how an act is defined. This act is usually one done by a practitioner in a patient-care giver interaction. The disease of chronic pain is complicated by multiple stakeholders including health care institutions, providers, families, insurers, pharmaceutical companies, government, and law enforcement. The simplicity of beneficence and nonmaleficence does not address the many spaces where acts that lead to good and acts that lead to the lack of good, both affecting a patient, will take place.

Beneficence and nonmaleficence in the treatment of chronic pain has been documented as the degree to which a provider is aware of a patient's pain and is dedicated the time and attention needed to treat that pain.[14] If we are willing to look at beneficence and nonmaleficence with a different lens, we will see issues of social justice that affect most everyone who has suffered from either the effects of chronic pain or the negative side effects of incomplete treatment.

The evidence is clear that a multidisciplinary approach to chronic pain management is more effective than individual treatment modalities.[15] This is true with health care in general. Any just treatment plan must consider what truly affects any person's or population's ability to realize health. Social justice as a principle requires us to consider contextual and structural inequities when allocating resources. Striving for equity with a social justice framework rather than for equality with a beneficence/nonmaleficence view reflects the commitment to allocating resources so that everyone has the capacity for health. A social justice framework asks us to rethink the factors that contribute to our health. Health behaviors should not be considered purely individual. Our behaviors are socially influenced, for example, by our access to healthy food and ability to exercise safely on our streets. The impact of our physical environment differs by where we are able to live, which is primarily socially determined. Social justice demands not simply that we provide proper advice to all patients regardless of context, but rather, that we tailor our advice to patients depending on their context (**Fig. 3**).

It is important to stress again that the only evidence-based management plans that have been shown to successfully treat chronic pain have been multidisciplinary approaches that consider social capital and societal influences.[15] The only way to

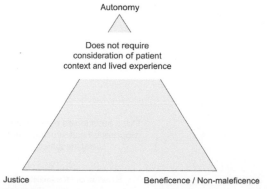

**Fig. 2.** Limitations of autonomy.

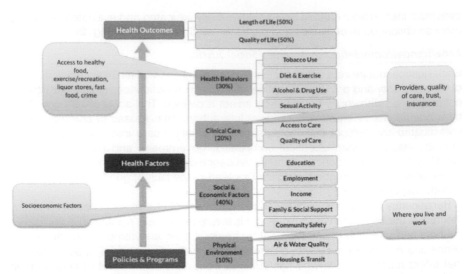

**Fig. 3.** County health rankings model. (The University of Wisconsin Population Health Institute. County Health Rankings & Roadmaps, 2022. www.countyhealthrankings.org.)

implement this approach in an equitable way is to make social justice a priority in the treatment of chronic pain. When treating a patient for chronic pain, a social justice approach would evaluate and react to positive and negative determinants of health affecting any patient's or population's relation to social and economic stability, mental health, physical environment, and health behaviors (**Fig. 4**).

People who experience chronic pain as well as social and structural inequities are experiencing social injustice. Social justice is only achieved through a realization and acceptance of social context; this is clearly evident in findings that show how persistent pain is not recognized, underestimated, and poorly managed in the marginalized populations. Multidisciplinary approaches to chronic pain management are rarely available to oppressed, marginalized populations. Social trauma, racism, lack of mental health resources, intentional poverty, and other challenges exaggerate the disparity in pain treatment. Knowing that these social injustices directly affect chronic

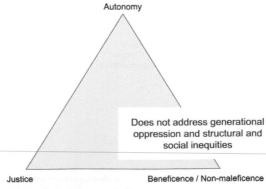

**Fig. 4.** Limitations of beneficence/nonmaleficence.

pain management requires that we address these injustices if we ever hope to treat manage chronic pain ethically.[16]

Medical education must share the specific experiences of affected patients and not only rely on the biomedical information. Personalized medicine need not be only about one's genome but include their lived experience. We also must acknowledge that there is inequity regarding mental health treatment[16] and that the ethical management of chronic pain requires a realization and correction of this clear health care disparity and social injustice. This approach will not only allow us to do good for patients and prevent us from doing harm, but also give us a roadmap to equitable care for everyone.

### Justice Becomes Solidarity

Within classic bioethics, justice refers primarily to distributive justice. This principle is meant to help prioritize cases and assure equality in the distribution of resources.[3] Prioritization and a goal of equality will not lead to ethical treatment within the complicated management of chronic pain. Without a clear lens to focus the stakeholders involved, the competing forces around business, pharmaceuticals, government, law enforcement, and health prevent the collective priority being allowing the patient capacity for health.

Solidarity should be added to our toolbox of principles. As a principle it binds 2 or more stakeholders together; it does not separate them into their disconnected corners of our bioethical conflict diagram. It is a principle that requires us to acknowledge that the social forces that led some of us to be particularly advantaged and set up for success are the same forces that have made it much more difficult for others. It is a principle that reinforces the fundamental healing bond between provider and patient, a bond that affirms that, as Levinas said, we each exist for the other.[17] It reminds us that, in the words of activist Lilla Watson, "If you have come here to help me, you are wasting your time. But if you have come because your liberation is bound up with mine, then let us work together."[18]

The invasion of business principles into medical care and its unintended negative consequences are most evident in current standard of care in the treatment of chronic pain.[4] Evidence has shown again and again the importance of a multidisciplinary approach and a strong mental health component, yet most chronic pain management teams use only a small portion of these evidence-based approaches.[19] We also must recognize that continued medical education, work-persons compensation, and medical school curricula are all significantly influenced by the industry that produces pain relieving medications.[20] Current litigation has begun to hold this industry accountable for how pain medications that we know are addictive were marketed.[21]

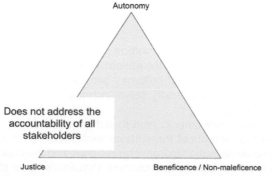

**Fig. 5.** Limitations of justice.

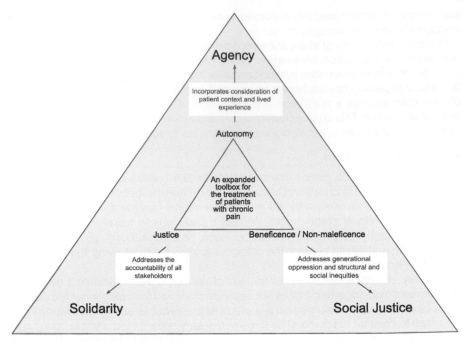

**Fig. 6.** The expanded bioethics toolbox.

Solidarity provides a roadmap to deal with the social injustices of generational trauma and oppression. Inequity across multiple social goods leads to bias and a disparity in care. Childhood adversity is an example of how a social context that greatly affects patients on an individual level is, itself, greatly affected by the generational disparity experienced by oppressed communities. These ongoing structural and social inequities worsen the impact childhood adversity has and sustains the cycle of disparity. This research is clear that communities affected by generational trauma manifesting as racism, sexism, and marginalization have less capacity for health and that breaking the cycle of generational oppression requires collaboration across multiple stakeholders.[22] Binding stakeholders together with similar, ethical goals would bring greater equity to the social construct of individuals' lived experience and a greater likelihood that more communities could experience a capacity for health[23]; this is especially evident with individuals and populations suffering from chronic pain (**Fig. 5**).

## SUMMARY

We believe that an expanded bioethics toolbox can encourage providers to think more broadly about the science of pain and the ethics of pain management. Adding the principles of agency, social justice, and solidarity provides a strong platform that helps providers and systems more ethically serve individuals and populations suffering from chronic pain (**Fig. 6**).

If we are to ethically treat chronic pain in patients and in populations, we must educate future practitioners about the embodiment of pain by patients, how practitioners experience patients suffering from chronic pain, and the importance of learning about a patient's lived experience and context. Practitioners, as stakeholders, must also embrace a broader sense of doing good and avoiding harm by advocating for socially just environments that provide individuals and communities capacity to experience more positive social and structural determinants of health. Practitioners and health care institutions need to stand with patients and populations most negatively affected by chronic pain and its consequences to hold all stakeholders with influence in the management of chronic pain accountable and keep the care of the patient central to patient care. Then, and only then, will we come closer to the ethical treatment of chronic pain.

## CLINICS CARE POINTS

- Consider your patient's experiences before they enter your examination room; broaden your understanding of "personal and social history" including individual, generational, and historical privilege, oppression, and trauma.

- Commit to providing true multidisciplinary care that is founded in the social environments in which people live their lives; broaden how you will see the provision of good care to include personalized structural and social determinants of health.

- Advocate for all stakeholders involved in the care and treatment of chronic pain to be held accountable to work toward individual and population capacity for health.

- Be part of a medical education curricula that uses the added urban bioethics principles of agency, social justice, and solidarity when caring for patients suffering from chronic pain.

## DISCLOSURE

The authors have nothing to disclose.

## REFERENCES

1. Post L, Blustein J, Gordon E, et al. Pain: ethics, culture, and informed consent to relief. J Law Med Ethics 1996;24:348–59.
2. Dahlhamer J, et al. Prevalence of chronic pain and high-impact chronic pain among adults—United States, 2016. MMWR Morb Mortal Wkly Rep 2018;67: 1001.
3. Beauchamp TL, Childress JF. Principles of biomedical ethics. 8th edition. New York: Oxford University Press; 2019. p. 13–5.
4. Loeser JD, Cahana A. Pain medicine versus pain management: ethical dilemmas created by contemporary medicine and business. Clin J Pain 2013;29(4):311–6.
5. Blustein J, Fleischman A. Urban bioethics: adapting bioethics to the urban context. Acad Med 2004;79(12):1198–202.
6. Gangas S. Sociologic theory and the capability approach. London (United Kingdom): Rutledge Taylor and Francis Group; 2020. p. 111–31.
7. Grisso T, Appelbaum PS. Assessing competence to consent to treatment: a guide for physicians and other health professionals. New York: Oxford University Press; 1998. p. 61–76.
8. Jonsen AR, et al. Clinical ethics. 5th edition. New York: McGraw-Hall; 2002. p. 57.
9. Felitti V, Anda R, Nordenberg D, et al. Relationship of childhood abuse and household dysfunction to many of the leading causes of death in adults - The adverse childhood experiences (ACE) study. Am J Prev Med 1998;14(4):245–58.
10. Brown D, Anda R, Tiemeier H, et al. Adverse childhood experiences and the risk of premature mortality. Am J Prev Med 2009;37(5):389–96.
11. Wade R, et al. Philadelphia ACE's Study. 2013. Available at: https://www.philadelphiaaces.org/philadelphia-ace-survey. Accessed November 20, 2021.

12. Spencer-Hwang R, Torres X, Valladares J, et al. Adverse Childhood Experiences among a Community of Resilient Centenarians and Seniors: Implications for a Chronic Disease Prevention Framework. Perm J 2018;22:17–146.
13. Douglas KR, Chan G, Gelernter J, et al. Adverse childhood events as risk factors for substance dependence: partial mediation by mood and anxiety disorders. Addict Behav 2010;35(1):7–13.
14. Pipien I. Bienfaisance et non-malfaisance dans les soins [Beneficence and non-maleficence in care]. Soins. 2018 Apr;63(824):51-54. French. doi: 10.1016/j.soin.2018.02.012. PMID: 29680141.
15. Turk DC, Okifuji A. Efficacy of multidisciplinary pain centers:antedote for anecdotes. Balliere's Clin Anesth 1998;12:103–19.
16. Wallace B, Varcoe C, Holmes C, et al. Towards health equity for people experiencing chronic pain and social marginalization. Int J Equity Health 2021;220:53.
17. Levinas E. Totality and infinity; an essay on exteriority. Pittsburgh (PA). Duquesne Univeristy Press. p. 31-102.
18. Meintjes B. Community-based psychosocial work to change the cycle of violence in post conflict areas. Social work in post-war and political conflict areas: examples from Iraqi-Kurdistan and beyond. 2019:111.
19. Portenoy R, Zeltzer L. Mayday Pain Report. A call to revolutionize chronic pain care in America: an opportunity in health care reform. New York. 2009:19.
20. Aronoff GM. FABPM Pain Treatment Centers at a Crossroads: a practical and conceptual reappraisal progress in pain research and management. Clin J Pain 1997;84–5.
21. Hodge JG Jr, Gostin LO. Guiding industry settlements of opioid litigation. Am J Drug Alcohol Abuse 2019;45(5):432–7.
22. Wade R Jr, Cronholm PF, Fein JA, et al. Household and community-level Adverse Childhood Experiences and adult health outcomes in a diverse urban population. Child Abuse Negl 2016;52:135–45.
23. Pachter LM, Lieberman L, Bloom SL, et al. Developing a Community-Wide Initiative to Address Childhood Adversity and Toxic Stress: A Case Study of The Philadelphia ACE Task Force. Acad Pediatr 2017;17(7S):S130–5.

# Guidelines and Policies
## Implications for Individual and Population Health

David T. O'Gurek, MD*, Menachem J. Leasy, MD

### KEYWORDS

• Guidelines • Overdose • Health equity • Trauma-informed care

### KEY POINTS

• Rising rates of opioid prescription for chronic pain occurring in conjunction with an evolving overdose crisis and rising rates of overdose deaths led to a significant focus on reducing opioid prescribing for chronic pain.

• Clinical practice guidelines (CPGs) provided guidance for the use of opioids in the treatment of chronic pain. Although guidelines specifically suggest they are no substitute for clinical judgment and the interpersonal patient-physician relationship, evidence of reduced opioid prescribing led to a growing number of policies and legislative efforts, prescriptive in the delivery of care.

• Misguided application of the guidelines into processes and policy created processes that lacked patient-centeredness and highlighted existing inequities in pain management care, rooted in systemic racism.

• Public health strategies that oversimplify a complex, multifaceted issue can produce intermediate or proxy outcomes that suggest improvements but do not have a meaningful impact on the health outcomes we are looking to change.

• A more holistic, trauma-informed approach that infiltrates both guidelines development as well as implementation will address psychosocial and physiologic factors that aid in prevention, treatment, and restorative efforts.

## INTRODUCTION

Strategies to address an ongoing and significant overdose crisis have led to evaluation to better understand the crisis. With an inflection point of rates of opioid prescribing for pain increasing in the 1990s and overdose deaths involving prescription opioids more than quadrupling from 1999 to 2019,[1] a focus for addressing the overdose crisis initially focused on prescription opioids. It has been well established that pharmaceutical

Department of Family and Community Medicine, Lewis Katz School of Medicine at Temple University, 1316 West Ontario Street, Philadelphia, PA 19140, USA
* Corresponding author.
E-mail address: David.O'Gurek@tuhs.temple.edu

Prim Care Clin Office Pract 49 (2022) 507–515
https://doi.org/10.1016/j.pop.2022.01.003
0095-4543/22/© 2022 Elsevier Inc. All rights reserved.

marketing directly to physicians, the most frequent source of prescription opioids for individuals who use opioids nonmedically,[2] during this time contributed to the increased prescription rates and concomitantly contributed to increased rates of overdose and overdose deaths.[3,4] In an effort to curb overdoses and overdose deaths, a growing number of guidelines for the management of pain as well as the use of opioids in the treatment of both acute and chronic pain developed. These guidelines serve as a foundational tool for physicians to gain appreciation around evidence-based principles for practice and served as part of a large public health strategy to address the overdose crisis. However, understanding the impacts of these guidelines, looking at both the intended and unintended consequences for both individual and population health is essential for the delivery of patient-centered care.

## CLINICAL PRACTICE GUIDELINES

Clinical practice guidelines (CPGs) serve as an evidence-based framework for making clinical decisions and supporting best practices in care. Informed by systematic reviews of evidence and assessments of benefits and harms, CPGs provide structured recommendations to optimize care. The National Academy of Medicine, formerly the Institute of Medicine (IOM), identifies 8 standards for developing trustworthy guidelines throughout the process that focuses on:

- Establishing transparency;
- Managing conflict of interest;
- Guideline development group composition;
- CPG-systematic review intersection;
- Establishing evidence foundations for and rating strength of recommendations;
- Articulation of recommendations;
- External review; and
- Updating.[5]

Despite unifying standards, there are variations in how different organizations use processes to meet these standards and therefore, critical review of guidelines is an important element of implementation into practice.

Guidelines addressing the management of pain including the use of opioids in the treatment of pain increasingly developed amidst the overdose crisis as increasing attention on prescription opioids. Professional organizations, states, and federal agencies either developed new or updated previous guidelines for opioid prescribing.[6-8] As a direct response to primary care physicians having concerns about opioid pain medication and the risks, reporting insufficient training in prescribing opioids[9] as well as belief that opioids had efficacy in managing pain,[10] the Centers for Disease Control and Prevention (CDC) developed a guideline for prescribing opioids for chronic pain in 2016.[11]

The CDC guideline was initially met with large acceptance including rapid uptake of the recommendations. Expansion upon the guideline with additional clinical tools were developed to facilitate implementation into practice[12] and the guideline received a high-quality rating from the ECRI Guidelines Trust Scorecard. Although opioid prescribing for chronic pain had been declining since 2012,[13] accelerated decrease occurred after the release of the CDC guideline.[14] Policymakers, attempting to curb the overdose crisis, translated guidelines into policy with government-directed opioid prescribing practices. By 2018, a majority of state Medicaid agencies reported implementing the guideline in their fee-for-service programs, and access to nonopioid pain medications was increased through passing of state laws.[15]

## CONTROVERSIES

CPG development around the utilization of opioids for pain management as well as legislation that directed pain management on the surface suggested that this was an efficacious strategy to curb overdoses and overdose deaths specifically from prescription opioids. When guidelines become policy, however, concerns arise. The guideline panel and processes were grounded in the NAM principles but were limited by the best available evidence at the time. For many individualized patient circumstances and questions that still remain around appropriate use of opioids, evidence is lacking and therefore the guideline cannot be appropriately extrapolated beyond its statements and intents to those situations. CPGs specifically express within their content that the guideline is voluntary and not prescriptive, unable to substitute for the relationship between clinician and patient that allows a deeper understanding of an individual's specific conditions and experiences. This ensures that patient-centered care occurs where the patient is an active participant in their care. This is disrupted particularly when legislative efforts go as far as imposing rigid dosing and duration limits.[16]

These policies and even translation to practice in health system policies and protocols have unfortunately been inconsistent with and been more restrictive than intended in the original guidelines. These inconsistencies including:

- Application of dosage ceilings and prescription duration guidance;
- Failure to appreciate the importance of patient involvement in decisions to taper or discontinue opioids;
- Barriers to diagnosis and treatment of opioid use disorder; and
- Impeded access to recommended comprehensive, multimodal pain care

were noted by a multidisciplinary expert panel that reviewed the influence of the core recommendations on practices and patients experiencing chronic pain.[17] Patients experiencing chronic pain, in many ways, felt abandoned by the system, targeted and stigmatized, and at times, incorrectly labeled as having opioid use disorder. When opioid use disorder was identified, strategies to ensure adequate treatment and provision of services were limited. Policies also did little, despite advocacy from the CDC, to improve access and reimbursement for services that would serve as part of multimodal pain care. In addition, the guideline focused specifically on chronic, noncancer pain; however, misapplication often affected patients with pain associated with cancer[17] and even acute sickle cell crises. The CDC guideline demonstrating restraint around the management of patients whose dose was above dose thresholds given limited evidence. Despite this, mandates and policies from insurers, health care systems, pharmacies, quality metric agencies, and contractors to the Centers for Medicare and Medicaid Services (CMS) used a dose threshold for distinguishing whether care was safe, payable, and even professional.[18] Concerns arose around whether patients who were forced to taper used other sources to both treat their pain as well as avoid potential withdrawal from underlying opioid dependence. Efforts to curb the negative effects of this led to the development of guidelines that would assist clinicians with patient-centered tapering strategies[19]; however, the harms created to individual patients as well as the community of patients experiencing chronic pain already broke significant trust with the system directed to protect and care for them.

The negative implications of inappropriate implementation of the guidelines amplified health inequities. A historically rooted and culturally reinforced system of discrimination,[20] structural racism serves as a foundational element to the inequities in chronic pain management. People of color have historically had less access to effective pain control, which is a disparity that continued to be evident with the emergence of the overdose crisis.[21,22] As guidelines developed, disparities in opioids were seen with studies showing patients identifying as black being more likely to receive drug testing,[23] being 2.1 and 3.3 times more likely than patients identifying as white to have therapy discontinued for respective cannabis and cocaine use,[24] and being at increased odds of dose reduction during pain treatment.[25] These disparities in monitoring, discontinuation, and dosing are not necessarily associated with worse outcomes nor are they a direct product of the guidelines themselves, but rather, importantly point to challenges within a system wrought with bias, explicit and implicit. They also highlight inequities within the same areas of concern raised by the multidisciplinary expert panel on guideline application. Furthermore, specific to access to treatment for opioid use disorder, history demonstrates the structural racism within our drug policy history, the war on drugs as a war on people of color, including racially targeted marketing strategies around buprenorphine[26] as well as disproportionate placement of buprenorphine programs in predominantly white and higher socioeconomic status neighborhoods.[27]

As part of the promise on guideline update and review as well as in response to criticisms that developed through misrepresentation of the guideline with implementation standards, the CDC began its work on updating their guideline in 2018, identifying appropriate partners and funding the Agency of Healthcare Research and Quality (AHRQ) to conduct systematic reviews. At this current time, the CDC is amidst a multi-year journey to update the guideline with the plan for an updated draft guideline to be available by early 2022 at which time it will seek comment from the public and specialty organizations to ensure diverse input to ensure a quality guideline.

## DISCUSSION

It is fair to say that every system is designed to get the results it gets. Limited understanding of the overdose crisis has led to oversimplification of the crisis with the CDC describing 3 waves:

- First wave rising in the 1990s with overdose deaths involving prescription drugs;
- Second wave beginning in 2010 with rapid increases in overdose deaths from heroin; and the
- Third wave beginning in 2013 with increasing overdoses resulting from synthetic opioids.[28]

Although this approach may characterize characteristics associated with rising rates of overdose and overdose death during more recent years, it fails to recognize past drug policy as well as structural racism that has underpinned US drug policy over time. This harmful history hovers as systems try to realign and create new approaches to addressing pain as well as substance use disorder; however, the experience suggests that white individuals are deserving of compassion and treatment, whereas our system previously and continually approaches people of color with suspicion and using a punitive approach.[29–32] Although well-intentioned, this 3-wave approach has at times directed attention toward symptoms with blame placed on pharmaceutical companies, prescribers, people who use drugs, organizations and hospital administrators, insurance providers, government regulators, and patients themselves. Focusing on the symptoms of the overall crisis distracts from addressing the root causes and process issues that each of these players faces on a regular basis around pain management.

Therefore, although the development of guidelines certainly is a feasible approach to delivering more evidence-based care, limited understanding of chronic pain among those who are using and interpreting the guideline may result in reduced prescriptions but does not necessarily translate to improving the quality of patient care for those experiencing chronic pain.[33] Shifting toward systems and policies that traditionally have taken a prohibitionist approach around substances have historically failed and resulted in increased use or evolution of the problem. And so, although the guidelines made their best effort using the evidence available, the expectation that a system with existing inequities, based on structural racism underfunding multimodal strategies around pain management, lacking appropriate education around the management of chronic pain, and lacking adequate treatment services for substance use disorder would squelch the overdose crisis through this approach was misguided.

A more appropriate public health approach requires a more holistic approach to addressing chronic pain both at the individual patient and population level. A holistic approach would balance patient rights, societal benefits of the treatment of chronic pain, the public health of the community, and the welfare of health care providers.[34] This does not necessarily translate to the absence of the creation of guidelines or translation of practice to policy; however, both must address systemic racism as well as trauma that is an essential component to managing chronic pain. These concepts are critical as well as interlinked. Trauma, broadly defined as experiences producing intense emotional pain, fear, or distress, often resulting in long-term physiologic and psychosocial consequences,[35] has broad impacts in chronic pain management[36,37] and particularly for those experiencing systemic trauma from structural inequalities.[38] Addressing equity will require data management and monitoring to evaluate inconsistencies in practice and application in a meaningful way to reduce system inequity. Focusing solely on the management of chronic pain as opposed to the care of the individual experiencing chronic pain narrows the impact and paves a path where opportunities to expand access to quality services get overlooked. The updates to the CDC guideline as well as further iterations may necessitate being more prescriptive around policy implications. In addition, policies need to adopt a trauma-informed approach, reflecting the 6 core principles of trauma-informed care including:

- Safety;
- Trustworthiness and transparency;
- Collaboration;
- Empowerment;
- Choice; and
- Intersectionality.[39]

Ensuring that these principles serve as the cornerstone for public health practice as well as policy enhances a health in all policies approach[40] to address complex problems that have a significant social and psychological overlay.[41] Although the process in creating a trauma-informed system is an ongoing and developmental journey, there are some simple strategies that physicians can use in practice to embrace these principles.[42] This holistic approach includes education, clinical care, and research components that alter the traditional approach and includes understanding prevention from a social and trauma-context, patient-centered treatment and management strategies, and restorative and rehabilitative services that ensure adequate access and covered to the quality, multidisciplinary services we know are essential to providing care to patients experiencing chronic pain.

## SUMMARY

The overdose crisis has stirred significant responses from several disciplines to develop public health strategies to reduce overdoses and overdose deaths; however, attempts at addressing symptoms of a multifaceted, complex problem can have negative implications on overall community and population health. The focus on the crisis occurring in waves with responses focused on curbing prescription opioids in the treatment of pain used the best available evidence at the time to create guidelines for practice. Rigid and overinterpretation of those guidelines led to policies that dictated care, used reduced opioid prescribing as a goal as opposed to improved overall quality, and that disrupted the physician-patient relationship, layering additional traumas onto a system already wrought with systemic racism, bias, and stigma.

With updates to guidelines and additional resources attempting to correct and control for the unintended consequences of these approaches, we must scrutinize our approaches and be inclusive in design, development, and monitoring to avoid replication of misapplication as well as perpetuation of stigma and inequity in management of chronic pain. Strategies that look to embrace trauma-informed principles will begin to transform culture within the systems that need structural changes to avoid producing the unsurprising results we currently get from them.

## CLINICS CARE POINTS

- Use a critical eye on evidence and strength of recommendations within guidelines as well as acknowledgment of guideline limitations and goals to not substitute for decision-making between patient and physician.

- Physicians should be aware of inequities in chronic pain management and use opportunities such as personal data review and implicit bias training in an effort to reduce disparities in chronic pain management.

- Physicians should increase educational efforts around chronic pain management and the intersectionality of trauma and components of trauma-informed care.

## DISCLOSURE STATEMENT

The authors have nothing to disclose.

## REFERENCES

1. Wide-ranging online data for epidemiologic research (WONDER). Atlanta, GA: CDC, national center for health statistics. 2020. Available at: http://www.wonder.cdc.gov. Accessed October 20, 2021.
2. International Narcotics Control Board. Narcotic drugs. 2016. Available at: https://www.incb.org/documents/Narcotic-Drugs/Technical-Publications/2016/Narcotic_Drugs_Publication_2016.pdf. Accessed October 20, 2021.
3. Larochelle MR, Zhang F, Ross-Degnan D, et al. Rates of opioid dispensing and overdose after introduction of abuse-deterrent extended-release oxycodone and withdrawal of propoxyphene. JAMA Intern Med 2015;175(6):978–87.
4. Hadland SE, Rivera-Aguirre A, Marshall BDL, et al. Association of pharmaceutical industry marketing of opioid products with mortality from opioid-related overdoses. JAMA Netw Open 2019;2(1):e186007.

5. Institute of Medicine (US). Committee on standards for developing trustworthy clinical practice guidelines. In: Graham R, Mancher M, Miller Wolman D, et al, editors. Clinical practice guidelines we can trust. Washington (DC): National Academies Press (US); 2011.

6. Chou R, Fanciullo GJ, Fine PG, et al. American pain society-american academy of pain medicine opioids guidelines panel. Clinical guidelines for the use of chronic opioid therapy in chronic noncancer pain. J Pain 2009;10:113–30.e22.

7. Washington State Agency Medical Directors' Group. AMDG 2015 interagency guideline on prescribing opioids for pain. Olympia, WA: Washington State Agency Medical Directors' Group; 2015. Available at: http://www.agencymeddirectors.wa.gov/guidelines.asp. Accessed October 20, 2021..

8. US Department of Veterans Affairs. VA/DoD clinical practice guidelines: management of opioid therapy (OT) for chronic pain. Washington, DC: US Department of Veterans Affairs; 2010. Available at: http://www.healthquality.va.gov/guidelines/Pain/cot. Accessed October 20, 2021.

9. Jamison RN, Sheehan KA, Scanlan E, et al. Beliefs and attitudes about opioid prescribing and chronic pain management: survey of primary care providers. J Opioid Manag 2014;10:375–82.

10. Wilson HD, Dansie EJ, Kim MS, et al. Clinicians' attitudes and beliefs about opioids survey (CAOS): instrument development and results of a national physician survey. J Pain 2013;14:613–27.

11. Dowell D, Haegerich TM, Chou R. CDC guideline for prescribing opioids for chronic pain – United States, 2016. MMWR Recomm Rep 2016;65(No. RR-1):1–49.

12. Dowell D, Haegerich TM. Changing the conversation about opioid tapering. Ann Intern Med 2017;167:208–9.

13. Guy GP, Zhang K, Bohm MK, et al. Vital signs: changes in opioid prescribing in the United States, 2006-2015. MMWR Morb Mortal Wkly Rep 2017;66(26):697–704.

14. Bohnert ASB, Guy GP Jr, Losby JL. Opioid prescribing in the United States before and after the centers for disease control and prevention's 2016 opioid guideline. Ann Intern Med 2018;169:367–75.

15. Centers for Medicare and Medicaid Services. CMCS informational bulletin: Medicaid strategies for non-opioid pharmacologic and non-pharmacologic chronic pain management. 2019. Available at: https://www.medicaid.gov/federal-policy-guidance/downloads/cib022219.pdf. Accessed October 20, 2021.

16. Dowell D, Haegerich T, Chou R. No shortcuts to safer opioid prescribing. N Engl J Med 2019;380(24):2285–7.

17. Kroenke K, Alford DP, Argoff C, et al. Challenges with implementing the Centers For Disease Control And Prevention opioid guideline: a consensus panel report. Pain Med 2019;20:724–35.

18. Kertesz SG, Gordon AJ, Manhapra A. Nonconsensual dose reduction mandates are not justified clinically or ethically: an analysis. J Law Med Ethics 2020;48(2):259–67.

19. Rich RR, Chou ER, Mariano A, Legreid Dopp R, Sullenger H. Burstin H and the Pain Management Guidelines and Evidence Standards Working Group of the Action Collaborative on Countering the U.S. Opioid Epidemic. 2020. Best Practices, Research Gaps, and Future Priorities to Support Tapering Patients on Long-Term Opioid Therapy for Chronic Non-Cancer Pain in Outpatient Settings. NAM Perspectives. Discussion Paper, National Academy of Medicine, Washington, DC.

20. Bailey ZD, Krieger N, Ageor M, et al. Structural racism and health inequities in the USA: evidence and interventions. Lancet 2017;389(10077):1453–63.

21. Becker WC, Starrels JL, Heo M, et al. Racial differences in primary care opioid risk reduction strategies. Ann Fam Med 2011;9(3):219–25.

22. Chen I, Kurz J, Pasanen M, et al. Racial differences in opioid use for chronic nonmalignant pain. J Gen Intern Med 2005;20(7):593–8.

23. Hausmann LR, Gao S, Lee ES, et al. Racial disparities in the monitoring of patients on chronic opioid therapy. Pain 2013;154(1):46–52.

24. Gaither JR, Gordon K, Crystal S, et al. Racial disparities in discontinuation of long-term opioid therapy following illicit drug use among black and white patients. Drug Alcohol Depend 2018;192:371–6.

25. Buonora M, Perez HR, Heo M, et al. Race and gender are associated with opioid dose reduction among patients on chronic opioid therapy. Pain Med 2019;20(8): 1519–27.

26. Netherland J, Hansen H. White opioids: pharmaceutical race and the war on drugs that wasn't. Biosocieties 2017;12(2):217–38.

27. Lagisetty PA, Ross R, Bohnert A, et al. Buprenorphine treatment divide by race/ethnicity and payment. JAMA Psychiatry 2019;76(9):979–81.

28. CDC. Three waves of opioid overdose deaths. Centers for disease control and prevention, national center for injury prevention and control, March 17, 2021. Available at: https://www.cdc.gov/opioids/basics/epidemic.html. Accessed October 30, 2021.

29. Bjerk D. Mandatory minimum policy reform and the sentencing of crack cocaine defendants: an analysis of the Fair Sentencing Act. J Empirical Legal Stud 2017; 14(2):370–96.

30. Bassett MT, Graves JD. Uprooting institutionalized racism as public health practice. Am J Public Health 2018;108(4):457–8.

31. Dasgupta N, Beletsky L, Ciccarone D. Opioid crisis: no easy fix to its social and economic determinants. Am J Public Health 2018;108(2):182–6.

32. Mendoza S, Rivera AS, Hansen HB. Re-racialization of addiction and the redistribution of blame in the white opioid epidemic. Med Anthropol Q 2019;33(2): 242–62.

33. Murray M, Stone A, Pearson V, et al. Clinical solutions to chronic pain and the opiate epidemic. Prev Med 2019;118:171–5.

34. Cohen SP, Baber ZB, Buvanendran A, et al. Pain management best practices from multispecialty organizations during the COVID-19 pandemic and public health crises. Pain Med 2020;21(7):1331–46.

35. Keesler JM. A call for the integration of trauma informed care among intellectual and developmental disability organizations. J Policy Pract Intell Disabil 2014; 11(1):34–42.

36. Felitti VJ, Anda RF, Nordenberg D, et al. Relationship of childhood abuse and household dysfunction to many of the leading causes of death in adults: the adverse childhood experiences (ACE) study. Am J Prev Med 1998;14(4):245–58.

37. Edwards RR, Dworkin RH, Sullivan MD, et al. The role of psychosocial processes in the development and maintenance of chronic pain. J Pain 2016;17(9 Suppl): T70–92.

38. McKenzie-Mohr S, Coates J, McLeod H. Responding to the needs of youth who are homeless: calling for politicized trauma-informed intervention. Child Youth Serv Rev 2012;34(1):136–43.

39. Elliott DE, Bjelajac P, Fallot RD, et al. Trauma-informed or trauma-denied: principles and implementation of trauma-informed services for women. J Community Psychol 2005;33(4):461–77.
40. Rudolph L, Caplan J, Ben-Moshe K, et al. Health in all policies: a guide for state and local governments. 2013. Available at: https://www.apha.org/~/media/files/pdf/factsheets/health_inall_policies_guide_169pages.ashx. Accessed October 21, 2021.
41. Bowen EA, Shaanta Murshid N. Trauma-informed social policy: a conceptual framework for policy analysis and advocacy. Am J Public Health 2016;106:223–9.
42. Leasy M, O'Gurek DT, Savoy ML. Unlocking clues to current health in past history: childhood trauma and healing. Fam Pract Manag 2019;26(2):5–10.

29. [...]

30. [...]

31. [...]

# Moving?

## Make sure your subscription moves with you!

To notify us of your new address, find your **Clinics Account Number** (located on your mailing label above your name), and contact customer service at:

Email: **journalscustomerservice-usa@elsevier.com**

**800-654-2452** (subscribers in the U.S. & Canada)
**314-447-8871** (subscribers outside of the U.S. & Canada)

Fax number: **314-447-8029**

**Elsevier Health Sciences Division**
**Subscription Customer Service**
**3251 Riverport Lane**
**Maryland Heights, MO 63043**

*To ensure uninterrupted delivery of your subscription, please notify us at least 4 weeks in advance of move.